Presenting Medical Statistics
from Proposal to Publication

PRESENTING MEDICAL STATISTICS
From Proposal to Publication
Second Edition

JANET L. PEACOCK

Professor of Medical Statistics,
Division of Health and Social Care Research,
Faculty of Life Sciences and Medicine,
King's College London, UK

SALLY M. KERRY

Reader in Medical Statistics,
Centre for Primary Care and Public Health,
Barts and the London School of Medicine and Dentistry,
Queen Mary University of London, UK

RAYMOND R. BALISE

Research Assistant Professor,
Department of Public Health Sciences, Division of Biostatistics,
University of Miami, USA
Stanford Cancer Institute and Department of Health Research and Policy,
Stanford, USA

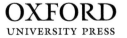

OXFORD
UNIVERSITY PRESS

OXFORD
UNIVERSITY PRESS

Great Clarendon Street, Oxford, OX2 6DP,
United Kingdom

Oxford University Press is a department of the University of Oxford.
It furthers the University's objective of excellence in research, scholarship,
and education by publishing worldwide. Oxford is a registered trade mark of
Oxford University Press in the UK and in certain other countries

First Edition published in 2007

Impression: 1

Published in the United States of America by Oxford University Press
198 Madison Avenue, New York, NY 10016, United States of America

British Library Cataloguing in Publication Data
Data available

Library of Congress Control Number: 2016960954

ISBN 978–0–19–877910–0

Printed and bound by
CPI Group (UK) Ltd, Croydon, CR0 4YY

This book is dedicated to the memory of
Graham Kerry

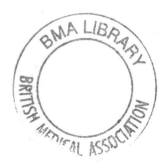

PREFACE TO THE SECOND EDITION

Much has happened since the 1st edition of *Presenting Medical Statistics from Proposal to Publication* was published in 2007. Most obviously, we have increased authors so that now we are three! We're so pleased that Ray Balise from the USA has joined us in making this 2nd edition bigger and better than the 1st and making it truly international. Ray had the inspiration to grow the book to include SAS, SAS University Edition, and R, as well as Stata and SPSS to meet the changing needs and practices of researchers. Our new edition retains the underlying flavour of the 1st in being example led, and showing how to undertake statistical analyses and how to report them. An added ingredient is the inclusion of code and datasets for all analyses shown in the book on our website (http://medical-statistics.info).

Readers of the 1st edition will notice that we don't include every analysis in all statistical packages–there wouldn't be space to do this. But instead we include one in the book, with each example being available on our website in all packages. We have updated where needed and added information on data protection and security in the USA as well as the UK. We have added a new chapter on meta-analysis.

We have retained the preface to the 1st edition as we still want to record our thanks to our many colleagues who have provided help in the form of data, examples, and/or general, much-appreciated support. In this edition we have some new people to thank: our heads of departments, who have supported us: Charles Wolfe (King's College London), Sandra Eldridge (Queen Mary University of London), and J. Sunil Rao (University of Miami) and also Phil Lavori and Alice Whittemore (Stanford). We thank Tim Peters, who kindly located and sent us the original data for figures 13.3 and 13.4, John Williams for permission to reproduce the pain meta-analyses, and Victoria Cornelius for the data dictionary example. Special thanks are needed for Justin Lock (King's), who spent many hours getting the screen shots into the right format for publishing and to Diane Morrison for help with production and proofing. We are grateful for all the support and patience shown to us by OUP staff, particularly Fiona Richardson.

Most of all we are grateful to our partners, Eric Peacock, Graham Kerry, and Lori Balise for all their encouragement and help. Very sadly, Graham died before we finished and so we dedicate this book to him.

PREFACE TO THE FIRST EDITION

The inspiration for this book has come from many years of designing, analysing, and reporting medical research studies ourselves, and giving advice to medical practitioners, researchers, and students. We have had a growing realization that presenting statistics is rarely straightforward. While there are many good medical statistics textbooks, these do not cover in detail the practical issues which many researchers grapple with at various stages of the research process, of how to present statistics. We have therefore tried to set in print the principles and ideas that we have assimilated over the years and which we have advised others to use too.

During our careers in medical research we have been privileged to work with many different colleagues, and the majority of examples in our book come from this rich source. We wish to thank our colleagues with whom we have collaborated in these research studies: Ross Anderson, Martin Bland, Maggie Bruce, Sandy Calvert, Franco Cappuccio, Iain Carey, Clare Chazot, Françoise Cluzeau, Derek Cook, Lyndsey Emmett, Anne Greenough, Phillip Hay, Sean Hilton, Alice Johnson, Samantha Johnson, Liz Limb, Neil Marlow, Louise Marston, Lesley Meyer, Pippa Oakeshott, Phil Peacock, Ruth Ruggles, Malcolm Stewart, Jane Scarlett, Andrew Steptoe, Glenn Stewart, David Strachan, Mark Thomas, and Christina Victor. We also wish to thank the many researchers and students who over the years have come to see us for statistical advice, and also those whose grant proposals and submitted papers we have reviewed. We have learnt so much through you, even though you never knew it!

We wish to express special thanks to Martin Bland, who has been an inspiration and encourager to us for many years and who has taught us so much about medical statistics. We are grateful to Martin and to Louise Marston for reading an earlier draft of our book and for making many helpful comments, although any errors or mistakes remain our own. We thank Phil Peacock for help in assembling the references. We are grateful for the support and patience shown us by the staff at Oxford University Press, especially when we were slow to deliver the manuscript. Finally, we wish to thank our long-suffering families, Eric, Jo, Rachelle, and Phil Peacock, and Graham, Paul, Philip, Sarah, and Sheila Kerry for their support throughout, and forbearance when we were at certain times constantly 'working on the book'.

JP & SK

FOREWORD

It has been said that experience is a great teacher, also that experience is what you needed five minutes before you got it. For the new researcher starting out on their first research project, either as a student, as a newly qualified professional, or simply out of curiosity, there is much to learn and many questions about how to proceed. Every research project is different; it is the nature of research. You are doing something which nobody has done before. Thus each research project is a journey into the unknown and on such a journey experience is the best guide.

What this book offers is some of the accumulated experience of three people who for a long time have been both carrying out research on questions in health and psychology and have been teaching others to do so. The experience they gained has been distilled into this book and presented in such a way as to be accessible to the new researcher. It is illustrated throughout with examples from studies carried out by the authors themselves.

Statistical analysis and statistical aspects of study design are one of the biggest obstacles, both to newcomers to research and, often, to those with considerable experience. Most researchers in healthcare are health professionals, whose training included only a little research methodology and statistics and whose primary concern is healthcare practice. Their primary focus, quite rightly, is on patients and other service users. Statistics can be an alien world.

It is now very easy to carry out statistical analysis. Computers continually increase in power and speed and statistical software continually expands in the variety of statistical procedures available. There are now many books and online resources which can guide the researcher through the choice of statistical method and readily available software which will carry out the chosen procedure. The gap, which this book bridges, is going from the output of the statistical program to the report for the reader. How do we take the output of a computer program and turn it into something which we can put into a dissertation or potential journal article?

The first edition of this book was a great step forward in helping researchers to do this. It covered two of the statistical programs, SPSS and Stata, which are widely used in health research. This second edition expands this by adding two more popular programs: SAS, widely used in the pharmaceutical industry, and R, often the choice in academia, not least because it is free. All of these programs have their advantages and often the choice is more to do with what is available and what previous experience the user has than their merits for a particular task. To keep the paper volume manageable, examples in all languages are available via the author's website (http://medical-statistics.info/presenting).

This second edition is expanded in other ways. A third author has joined the team, extending the range of experience on which they can draw and widening the geographical range in which this experience has been gained. The authors of this book are very experienced teachers and communicators of statistics in health and related fields. I worked with Janet Peacock and Sally Kerry for many years. Together we taught thousands of students and produced 22 published papers and a book. I trust them completely to explain with clarity. The addition of Raymond Balise can only make their collaboration even better.

Statistics, like most subjects, does not stand still. It has responded to the desire for evidence-based practice by adding a new topic: meta-analysis. Since the first edition was published, the number of meta-analyses appearing in journals has increased rapidly and their importance for the new researcher has increased also. Now, I find that many students are doing systematic reviews and meta-analyses as part of, or the entirety of, their dissertations and theses. More established researchers are being asked to carry out a systematic review and meta-analysis before embarking on a new study, then to repeat this including the results of the new study when completed. The inclusion of this topic is very welcome.

The size and complexity of the studies reported in the major journals increases correspondingly, with ever more intricate statistical analyses being presented. To join this world at any level can be very daunting. With this book beside you, at least some of the obstacles will be easier to cross.

Martin Bland
Emeritus Prof. of Health Statistics
University of York

CONTENTS

1 Introduction 1

2 Introduction to the research process 4

3 Writing a research protocol 22

4 Writing up a research study 39

5 Introduction to presenting statistical analyses 48

6 Single group studies 64

7 Comparing two groups 72

8 Analysing matched or paired data 97

9 Analysing relationships between variables 114

10 Multifactorial analyses 134

11 Survival analysis 161

12 Presenting a randomized controlled trial 173

13 Presenting a meta-analysis 195

References 219
Index 223

DETAILED CONTENTS

1 Introduction   **1**
  1.1 The use of statistics in research   1
  1.2 Presenting medical statistics   1
  1.3 This book   2
  1.4 Final words   3

2 Introduction to the research process   **4**
  2.1 Defining the research question   4
  2.2 Writing a research protocol   5
  2.3 Data collection   6
  2.4 Transferring the data to computer   7
  2.5 Data checking and cleaning   14
  2.6 Using computer packages   16
  2.7 Record keeping   16
  2.8 Presenting results   20
  2.9 When to seek help from a statistician   20

3 Writing a research protocol   **22**
  3.1 The development cycle   22
  3.2 Title   22
  3.3 Aims of the research study   23
  3.4 Primary and secondary aims   24
  3.5 Study design   24
  3.6 Sample size calculations   24
  3.7 Plan of statistical analysis   34
  3.8 Required approval for research   34
  3.9 When applications fail   38

4 Writing up a research study   **39**
  4.1 Introduction   39
  4.2 Contents of each section of the report   39
  4.3 Special circumstances   46

5 Introduction to presenting statistical analyses   **48**
  5.1 Introduction   48
  5.2 Presenting numerical data   48

5.3	Beginning the results section	49
5.4	Describing the results of the recruitment process	49
5.5	Assessing non-response bias	51
5.6	Presenting the results for different media	52
5.7	Drawing up a profile of a group of subjects	56
5.8	Drawing graphs	56
5.9	Using text to refer to tables and graphs	57
5.10	Presenting categorical data	58
5.11	Presenting continuous data	58

6 Single group studies   **64**

6.1	Introduction	64
6.2	Prevalence studies	64
6.3	Presenting the results of prevalence studies	65
6.4	Screening and diagnostic studies: Sensitivity and specificity	66
6.5	Presentation of sensitivity and specificity	67
6.6	Comment on results	67
6.7	Screening studies for rare conditions	68
6.8	Extensions to sensitivity and specificity	70
6.9	Further reading	70

7 Comparing two groups   **72**

7.1	Introduction	72
7.2	Graphical presentation of continuous unpaired data	72
7.3	Continuous unpaired data: The two-sample *t* test	75
7.4	Mann–Whitney *U* test	79
7.5	Comparing two proportions	82
7.6	Further reading	96

8 Analysing matched or paired data   **97**

8.1	Introduction	97
8.2	Continuous paired data: The paired *t* test	98
8.3	Non-Normal data	102
8.4	Matched case-control data	104
8.5	Matched cohort data	108
8.6	Further reading	113

9 Analysing relationships between variables   **114**

9.1	Introduction	114
9.2	Correlation	114
9.3	Regression	124
9.4	Further reading	132

10 **Multifactorial analyses**   **134**
   10.1 Introduction   134
   10.2 One-way analysis of variance   136
   10.3 Multiple regression   140
   10.4 Logistic regression   149

11 **Survival analysis**   **161**
   11.1 Introduction   161
   11.2 Kaplan–Meier estimates of survival rates   165
   11.3 The logrank test   165
   11.4 Cox regression   166
   11.5 Further reading   172

12 **Presenting a randomized controlled trial**   **173**
   12.1 Introduction to the CONSORT statement   173
   12.2 The CONSORT checklist   174
   12.3 Intention-to-treat analysis   189
   12.4 Cluster randomized trials   191
   12.5 Reporting guidelines for other study designs   193

13 **Presenting a meta-analysis**   **195**
   13.1 Introduction to systematic reviews and meta-analysis   195
   13.2 Statistics and meta-analysis   200
   13.3 The PRISMA statement   200
   13.4 Reviewing meta-analyses   216
   13.5 Further reading   217

References   219
Index   223

CHAPTER 1

Introduction

1.1 **The use of statistics in research** *1*
1.2 **Presenting medical statistics** *1*
1.3 **This book** *2*
1.4 **Final words** *3*

1.1 The use of statistics in research

Medical statistics is the discipline that provides the tools to turn numerical information into evidence. This evidence might be for the cause of a disease or for the effectiveness of an intervention. The advent of evidence-based medicine has led to a greater demand for such research evidence.

The majority of researchers in medicine and the healthcare professions now use statistics in their research. It is easier than ever before for researchers to do their own statistical analyses using one of the many available statistical programs with their user-friendly interfaces. This is probably a mixed blessing.

On the positive side, researchers can now be independent and no longer have to rely on finding a friendly statistician to do analyses for them. The downside is that, because statistical programs are easy to use, it is equally easy to do the wrong analysis. Even if the right analysis is performed, the programs often produce lots of output which tends to contain some relevant and some irrelevant results. Selecting the appropriate results from such output is not always straightforward. In addition, statistical programs, though very sophisticated, do not generally tell the user if a particular analysis is valid or not.

1.2 Presenting medical statistics

Research is conducted as part of a search for more knowledge. For the most part, the researcher fully intends to share newly gained knowledge with others so that they can benefit from the findings, in future research, in professional practice, or both. However, the sharing of research findings sometimes causes difficulty. The presentation of statistical information is not straightforward, and yet inadequate presentation will fail to communicate the relevant information and may even communicate misleading or incorrect information.

The EQUATOR group (Altman et al. 2008) seeks to promote clear reporting of research findings for randomized trials (CONSORT: Shultz et al. 2010) and observational studies 'to improve the reliability of medical publications by promoting transparent and accurate reporting of health research'. The EQUATOR group argues that the reader must be able to understand all parts of the study process and that full and transparent presentation is needed to achieve this. It is clear that good presentation skills are crucial in all areas of evidence-based practice so that other practitioners can critically assimilate and interpret evidence and then turn that evidence into better practice.

1.3 **This book**

This book describes the presentation of required statistical information through the entire research process, from the development of the research proposal, through analysing the data, to writing up the results. The term 'statistical information' includes the description of the study design, the calculation of sample size, and data processing, as well as data analysis and reporting of results. *Presenting Medical Statistics* is written for researchers in medicine and in professions allied to medicine.

The first part of the book describes the research process and discusses how to write a research protocol and how to report the statistical aspects in regulatory and ethical approval applications. General guidelines are given on writing up a study for different media, such as a web page, a journal paper, a report, a dissertation or thesis, or an oral or poster presentation. The second part of the book illustrates how to present different analyses, going from simple descriptive to more complex analyses, such as Cox regression. Throughout the book we use examples and analyses from real research, mostly our own.

Examples are given of how to present statistical information, for a proposal, a paper, or a report, usually in a concise format that it is appropriate for a shorter report or journal paper but that can easily be expanded to suit a longer document, such as a dissertation or thesis. We show how the methods and results sections can be written and also give some discussion points to show how the interpretation of statistical findings might feed into the discussion section.

1.3.1 **Statistical analyses and software**

The main analyses in the book are performed in SAS 9.4, SAS University Edition, R version 3.1.2, Stata 13, and SPSS v22, five of the most popular statistical programs available. For most analyses only one output is shown in the book but all outputs, and the code needed to generate them, are available on our website http://medical-statistics.info/presenting alongside the complete datasets. While not every package can render every plot without a huge amount of work, whenever reasonable we have provided instructions for generating the graphics and tables.

For each figure there is a colour graphic showing the code, and below it the code is shown in easy-to-copy text format. SAS University Edition features some menus but some analyses can only be done using code. SPSS uses menus. The website provides for these options.

Some sample size calculations are done in Epi-Info and G*Power; both packages are free and can be downloaded from the web.

1.3.2 **Reporting results**

We show how the results from statistical programs can be translated into text or tables for inclusion in a written document, indicating which particular results in an output are relevant and giving an example of how they can be presented and described.

Where a published study is used, the reference is provided so that readers can look at it if they wish. Sometimes the original analyses are shown in a simplified or reduced form where, for example, many variables had been included but only a few are needed to illustrate the point we wish to make.

1.3.3 References

Books and journal articles are listed in short-form in the text but in full in the reference section. Websites are listed in full as they appear. Since most examples are drawn from our own research, where example data are described further in a paper (e.g. Peacock et al. 1991), we give the full reference, saying 'For further information see Peacock JL, Bland JM, Anderson HR. Effects on birthweight of alcohol and caffeine consumption in smoking women. *J Epidemiol Community Health* 1991; 45:159–163.'

1.3.4 Using this book

The boxes found alongside the detailed descriptions are there to help readers, and contain various types of material for quick access—helpful tips, examples, summaries, and information. In addition, each chapter has a summary box at the end highlighting the main points covered in the chapter.

Presenting Medical Statistics is not a textbook but a practical reference book. Few readers will read straight through the book but most will dip into particular sections and the linked web pages as needed. While the 'information' boxes indicate both the theoretical and the practical issues to consider when reporting statistics, throughout the book there are references to medical statistics textbooks and other information for fuller details. These references are not exhaustive; the books are those that we have on our bookshelves and with which we are familiar as well as those we have written ourselves. There are undoubtedly many excellent statistics books that we have not been able to mention and we apologize for this. The software that we have used is only a sample of all that is available. Researchers who use programs other than those included in this book will still find much useful information here.

The main steps in setting up a research study are set out, as are all of the analyses commonly used, as well as some of the more complex ones. As software and fashions change, different analyses become more widespread and there are certain to be some omissions. The principles given in this book will guide researchers in presenting statistical material in all parts of the research process with different study designs and different analyses.

When making practical suggestions for presenting statistical information, varying formats for presenting graphs, tables, and results are used in different parts of the book, reflecting the real world. Often, there is no single 'right' way to present findings, but there are often unhelpful or wrong ways.

Chapters of the book frequently refer to other sections for other examples or where more explanation is required. However, each chapter is relatively self-contained, and some repetition or reinforcement of material is therefore unavoidable.

1.4 Final words

We will add additional new material to the web from time to time so check it out. All analyses and presentations have been checked but it is always possible that errors have slipped through. If you find any errors or mistakes in this book, please tell us via janet. peacock@kcl.ac.uk and we will post corrections on the web (http://medical-statistics. info).

CHAPTER 2

Introduction to the research process

2.1 **Defining the research question** *4*

2.2 **Writing a research protocol** *5*

2.3 **Data collection** *6*

2.4 **Transferring the data to computer** *7*

2.5 **Data checking and cleaning** *14*

2.6 **Using computer packages** *16*

2.7 **Record keeping** *16*

2.8 **Presenting results** *20*

2.9 **When to seek help from a statistician** *20*

2.1 Defining the research question

Often research begins with a general question in the researcher's mind, such as 'I wonder why . . . ?' or 'I wonder if . . .?' perhaps arising from an observation, as illustrated in box 2.1. Such enquiry is an essential prerequisite to the research process but is not sufficient to design a study.

A research study needs to have a specific question which the researcher wishes to answer. This might take the form of a simple question, such as 'What is the prevalence of asthma in the UK?' Alternatively, the research question may be a hypothesis to test, such as 'Is the prevalence of asthma increasing?' In a study testing a hypothesis the researcher is looking for evidence for or against this hypothesis so that he can make an informed decision as to whether or not it is likely to be true.

However, even these questions are not sufficiently defined. The first example appears straightforward until we consider what is meant by 'asthma' and in which age groups we are interested. We then might tighten up our question to 'What is the prevalence of doctor-diagnosed asthma in adults in the UK?' Similar issues arise in the second example. We need to know what is meant by 'an increase' and determine the time period. Thus, we might refine our question to ask 'Has the prevalence of doctor-diagnosed asthma in adults increased in the past 10 years?' Other examples are shown in box 2.2.

These examples illustrate the importance of tightly defining our research question. Once we have a research question, then the required study design is easier to decide upon. In addition, the research question needs to be one that can be answered. For example, a published

---

Box 2.1 An observation   *EXAMPLE*

It was observed that several patients receiving treatment for hypertension reported improvement in migraine while taking lisinopril. This led to a randomized trial to address the following research questions.

♦ *Does lisinopril reduce the number of days affected by migraine, number of hours with headache, and number of days with headache?*

♦ *What is the reduction in blood pressure when lisinopril is prescribed to patients with normal blood pressure?*

For further information see Schrader H, Stovner LJ, Helde G, Sand T, Bovim G. Prophylactic treatment of migraine with angiotensin converting enzyme inhibitor (lisinopril): randomised, placebo controlled, crossover study. BMJ 2001; 322:19–22

---

study sought to determine whether an episode of a UK TV programme, *Casualty*, which involved a suicide, caused an increase in suicide rates in the population (Hawton et al. 1999). The researchers reported that an increase in the suicide rate was observed, but they concluded that they could not say if the episode actually caused the increase. That question is not answerable.

2.2 **Writing a research protocol**

A research protocol is a formal document outlining the proposed study and is an essential part of the study design and conduct. It starts with the research question, discusses what is already known about the topic, and explains how the proposed study will further knowledge. It then describes the study design and provides details of how the study will be conducted, including a plan for any statistical analysis.

There are few occasions in medical research where a protocol is unnecessary, and so it is recommended that researchers always write one. The length and extent of detail required will vary—for example, a protocol for a small student project will be shorter than one needed for a multi-centre clinical trial where detailed instructions for conducting the study are essential to maintain uniformity. These points are summarized in boxes 2.3 and 2.4, and full details on writing a protocol are given in chapter 3.

Box 2.2 Examples of specific research questions   *EXAMPLE*

♦ What is the prevalence of doctor-diagnosed asthma in adults in the UK?

♦ Has the prevalence of doctor-diagnosed asthma in adults increased in the past 10 years?

♦ What is the prevalence of chlamydia infection among asymptomatic women attending for cervical smear tests in inner-city General Practices in the UK?

♦ Is miscarriage at less than 16 weeks associated with bacterial vaginosis infection diagnosed before 10 weeks gestation?

Box 2.3 Reasons for writing a research protocol	*SUMMARY*

Scientific Focuses ideas about the research question, sets it in the context of what is already known.

Feasibility Sample size calculations and a statistical plan help to ensure that aims can be achieved.

Monitoring Provides a timetable and plan to monitor the progress of the study.

Organizational Provides the basis for applications for funding and ethical approval.

Aide memoire For writing up the study at a later date.

2.3 Data collection

The collection of data—what is actually collected and the format it is in—is obviously related to the study protocol. It is important to know in advance what we are going to do with the data in order to ensure that it is collected in the right format. For example, if we want to calculate mean age in a study group then we should record actual age rather than age in 10-year age bands. When collecting original data, it is not always easy to know exactly which data to collect. Some of the issues surrounding this are discussed in box 2.5.

It may be possible to answer a research question using existing data (box 2.6). However, great care must be taken to understand the social construction of the data, that is, the context and purpose for which the data were collected. These factors may have affected the data completeness and accuracy and led to bias in the data values. For example, data used for charging may have a tendency to inflate the severity of a condition. Guidelines for the reporting of routinely collected data were published by the EQUATOR Network (http://www.equator-network.org). The quality of pre-existing data will also need to be inspected thoroughly. While many systems have checks on the limits of individual values, making it impossible to enter a neonate's weight as 45 kg, for example, such systems rarely use even the most rudimentary logic checks to examine two things at once. For example, research databases and hospital electronic medical record systems routinely contain men with ovarian cancer, and women with prostate problems.

Box 2.4 Summary of a research protocol	*SUMMARY*

- Title
- Abstract
- Purpose of the study; aims
- Background
- Study design
- Justification for sample size
- Plan of statistical analysis
- Ethical issues
- Costs
- Timetable
- Personnel

| Box 2.5 Beware of collecting too much data | *INFORMATION* |

Consider these questions:

- Why are you collecting it?
- Will it actually be analysed?
- Who will be in charge of quality control on each question?

Disadvantages of long questionnaires:

- They may discourage people from taking part and so lower the response rate
- Questions may be answered less carefully
- Data processing time may be increased and results may be delayed
- They may lead to multiple hypothesis tests which increase the chance of spurious significance
- Time and money may be wasted

However it is important to collect what you do need as it may be difficult to get it later.

2.4 Transferring the data to computer

2.4.1 Coding

The researcher needs to decide how the data are to be recorded in a computer. All analysis packages make a distinction between numeric and character data. Character data can consist of letters and/or numbers but will not be used for calculations; numeric data contain only numbers and decimal places, with a minus sign for negative values. Numeric data are typically formatted to include characters to indicate pounds or dollars, as well as commas or decimals between the thousands digits, but behind the scenes this formatting is stripped away. As you load data into your analysis tool, be sure to check that it is identifying the data type correctly.

| Box 2.6 Points concerning the use of existing datasets | *INFORMATION* |

- Can be cheaper and quicker than collecting new data
- Time must be spent doing quality control on the data
- The research question needs to be defined and researched in the same way as for a primary study
- A clear analysis plan is needed to avoid overanalysing the data
- The dataset may not contain all the necessary information to answer the new question
- Analysis of data that has been collected for another purpose is sometimes referred to as **secondary analysis**

Consider the purpose for which the data were collected and how this might affect the data values.

Because they are so hard to clean up, code, and analyse, fill-in-the-blank questions are best avoided if possible. For example, a fill-in-the-blank question such as 'Country of Birth' could result in the following answers: USA, United States, U.S.A., America, Texas, etc. Instead, likely choices should be listed as tick boxes and then another option should be provided with a fill-in-the-blank for the remaining 'other' answers.

Before non-numeric data from a questionnaire or data collection form are entered onto a computer, the responses need to be coded. That is, a unique number should be assigned to each possible response to facilitate statistical analysis. Some statistical packages will analyse data which are non-numeric but in general it is easier to assign a different number to the different responses. For example, in figure 2.1, the question 'When did you have rhinitis?' can be answered with 'Dry season' (=1), 'Wet season' (=2), 'Anytime' (=3), or 'Never' (=4). Ideally, these code numbers should be stored as character values to avoid the possibility of doing calculations, such as computing the average season, on such categorical data, which would be nonsensical.

We suggest coding yes/no questions as numeric data with 1 for yes and 0 for no. Using such a scheme makes it easy to calculate the total number and percentage of 'yes' responses.

Keep in mind that the response to a 'choose one' question is a single answer but a 'tick all that apply' question is actually a series of yes/no questions and will need to be coded as many separate questions in a database. The coding for a single question and for multiple choice questions is shown in box 2.7. If data need coding, it can be useful to leave room on

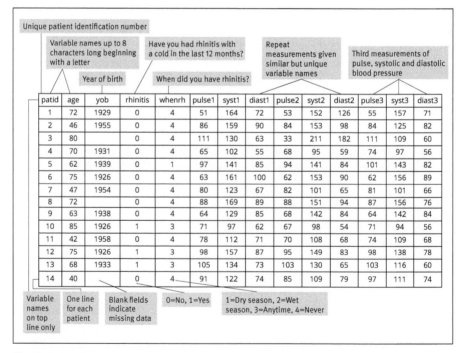

Figure 2.1 Portion of a spreadsheet showing data collected from participants in a screening survey (example)

the data collection form or questionnaire for the codes to be added by the researcher after the form has been returned. These are sometimes in a column down the right hand side of forms, labelled 'For office use only'.

In general, data should be kept ungrouped if possible. For instance, asking patients for their actual age at diagnosis is preferable to age at diagnosis in 10-year categories, since keeping the data ungrouped retains all the information and gives maximum flexibility for analysis now and later. Of course, asking subjects to recall in great detail can lead to a false sense of precision. Respondents may not know the exact age of ovarian cancer for an aunt but they may know ±5 years. In such cases it is wise to ask for approximate age and then ask for the approximate precision as ±1 year, ±5 years, ±10 years, etc.

2.4.2 Missing data

Missing data are undesirable in any study. It is important to be able to distinguish between data which are missing because the subject failed to respond (i.e. missed the question completely) and where the answer is 'Don't know'. For example, if question 1 in box 2.7 does not include the 'Never' category, it is unclear what it means when a patient doesn't tick any box. It could mean that they never had rhinitis or they skipped the question. Similarly, every 'Yes' box on a questionnaire should have a corresponding 'No'. Ticking 'Patient had

---

Box 2.7 Coding single and multiple questions   *EXAMPLE*

1. The following **single question** was asked in the screening survey (see figure 2.1)

When did you have rhinitis? *(Please tick one answer)*
- ❒ Dry season   (=1)
- ❒ Wet season   (=2)
- ❒ Anytime   (=3)
- ❒ Never   (=4)

The question would be coded 1, 2, 3, or 4, according to the single answer given. Without choice 4 it is unclear if the subject never had rhinitis or failed to answer the question.

2. The following **multiple question** was asked in a study of patients with low back pain.

What did you expect from your consultation with your GP? *(Please tick all that apply)*
- ❒ Prescription
- ❒ Advice
- ❒ Referral for x-ray
- ❒ Referral to consultant
- ❒ Certificate off work

Although this is one question each person may tick a number of options. This needs to be entered as five separate variables each coded as 'no' or 'yes', which could be entered as 0 or 1.

an adverse drug reaction' on a case report form indicates the subject had an adverse event but if the box is not ticked it is unclear if the patient had no adverse event or if the box was missed. Rather than use a blank field to indicate a completely missing response, it is usually preferable use a code which is not a valid code for the other answers.

Many researchers use a 'similar' but impossible code number to indicate missing values—for example, if age at HIV transmission is coded as −1 for a patient who did not know when they were infected, or −9 is coded for 'refused to answer', a researcher analysing the data in the middle of the night before a deadline may calculate the average age with those codes included and not notice that anything is amiss. Instead, it's far safer to use values that are clearly out of range, such as missing age coded as −1,000,000 or −9,000,000, so that any averages computed will be clearly noticeable as impossible, even at 4 a.m., and the problem will be noted, saving the researcher a correction/retraction.

2.4.3 Documentation

When data are coded, a data dictionary describing the meaning of each code (also known as a coding schedule) should be kept for future reference. A data dictionary should contain the original questions from the questionnaire, a short easy-to-type name for these questions, called the 'variable name', the variable label, the data type, e.g. date, integer, etc., and values, e.g. 1 = yes, 0 = no for numeric variables. If appropriate it should also state the minimum and maximum possible values (e.g. age at first childbirth, 9–60 years) and the likely values (e.g. age at first childbirth likely between 16 and 45). Including the inner and outer bounds on numeric variables in the dictionary makes it easy to document and automate quality control checks for 'expected' versus 'odd' versus 'impossible' values. Table 2.1 shows an extract of a data dictionary as an example.

Many longitudinal research studies make small changes to questionnaires part way through the project as new questions are added. For this reason, the questionnaire should always state the version number so that, if the database for a project indicates that a subject took, for example, a questionnaire's version 2.0, and a question of interest didn't appear until version 2.1, then that would explain certain missing data.

2.4.4 Protecting patients' information

It is important for the data collection forms to include a unique identifier for each subject so that, if needed, the computer records can later be compared with the original written forms, and that multiple forms for the same subject, perhaps collected at different times, can be matched up. The key that matches the unique identifier to the participant's name needs to be kept securely in a place that is different from that where the data collection forms are kept. To maintain patient confidentiality the patient identifier should not be a name or hospital number which might reveal the subject's identity. Box 2.8 lists elements considered Protected Health Information (PHI) in the United States. Researchers in other countries may also find this list useful in considering what constitutes patient identifiable data. We advise such elements not be stored in the data collection forms and research database unless specialist advice has been sought over appropriate data security measures.

While it requires a computer security expert for its initial set-up, REDCap (http://www.project-redcap.org) is an excellent, user-friendly, free, web-based database for collecting and storing research data, including PHI. REDCap allows patients or researchers

			Table 2.1 Extract of a data dictionary		EXAMPLE
Visit	Page	Variable name	Label	Data type	Values
vis1	1	studyid	Study ID	scale	integer
vis1	1	dob	date of birth	date	dd/mm/yyyy
vis1	1	dov1	date of first visit	date	dd/mm/yyyy
vis1	1	bq1v1	asthma start (age in years)	scale	integer
vis1	1	bq2v1	reliever start (age in years)	scale	integer
vis1	1	bq3v1	preventer start (age in years)	scale	integer
vis1	1	bq4v1	months asthma worse_Dec-Feb	nominal	1 = yes, 0 = no
vis1	1	bq5v1	months asthma worse_Mar-May	nominal	1 = yes, 0 = no
vis1	1	bq6v1	months asthma worse_Jun-Aug	nominal	1 = yes, 0 = no
vis1	1	bq7v1	months asthma worse_Sep-Nov	nominal	1 = yes, 0 = no
vis1	1	bq8v1	months asthma worse_ nospecifmonth	nominal	1 = yes, 0 = no
vis1	1	bq9v1	triggers_weather	nominal	1 = yes, 0 = no
vis1	1	bq10v1	triggers_pollen	nominal	1 = yes, 0 = no
vis1	1	bq11v1	triggers_emotions	nominal	1 = yes, 0 = no
vis1	1	bq12v1	triggers_fumes	nominal	1 = yes, 0 = no
vis1	1	bq13v1	triggers_dust	nominal	1 = yes, 0 = no
vis1	1	bq14v1	triggers_pets	nominal	1 = yes, 0 = no
vis1	1	bq15v1	triggers_cold/flu	nominal	1 = yes, 0 = no
vis1	1	bq16v1	triggers_cigarette smoke	nominal	1 = yes, 0 = no
vis1	1	bq17v1	triggers_foods/drinks	nominal	1 = yes, 0 = no
vis1	1	bq18v1	triggers_soaps/sprays/detergent	nominal	1 = yes, 0 = no
vis1	1	bq19v1	triggers_exercise	nominal	1 = yes, 0 = no
vis1	1	bq20v1	triggers_other things	nominal	1 = yes, 0 = no
vis1	1	bq20v1a	triggers_other things, specify	string	250 characters

to fill out online questionnaires or use data-entry forms on desktop, laptop, and tablet computers with only a secure internet connection through their web browser. The data are stored securely, complete with an audit trail to keep track of who did what to the data and when. REDCap exports into SAS, R, Stata, SPSS, and Excel. It has exceptionally good controls to protect the identities of subjects by limiting which variables are shown and exported and it can systematically modify dates so that dates of medical service are obscured but the values can still be used for analyses that need dates, such as survival analyses.

For researchers carrying out randomized trials in the UK we recommend contacting a registered Clinical Trial Unit at an early stage in the development of the protocol, who may be able to provide a suitable secure database with audit trails (http://www.ukcrc-ctu.org.uk). A Clinical Trials Unit will usually also provide statistical support in addition to randomization, advice on data management, and advice regarding the regulatory requirements. Statistical support, randomization, database set-up, and data management usually require costing and are commonly included as items in a funding application.

Box 2.8 Protected Health Information (PHI)   *INFORMATION*

The following elements are considered PHI in the US:

* Names
* Geographical identifiers smaller than a state (note that the 1st three digits of the zip code may be acceptable if the zip code region contains >20,000 people)
* Dates directly related to an individual
* Phone, fax numbers
* Email addresses
* Social security numbers
* Medical record numbers
* Health insurance beneficiary numbers
* Account numbers
* Certificate/license numbers
* Vehicle identifiers and serial numbers, including license plate numbers
* Device identifiers and serial numbers
* Web Uniform Resource Locators (URLs)
* Internet Protocol (IP) address numbers
* Biometric identifiers, including finger, retinal, and voice prints
* Full face photographic images and any comparable images
* Any other unique identifying number, characteristic, or code

https://www.hhs.gov/hiPaa/for-professionals/privacy/special-topics/de-identification/

Data can be entered directly onto a computer by using a spreadsheet (see figure 2.1). Each subject should have one line on the spreadsheet, and each unique question should have one column. It is critically important that each column contains only one type of information. For example, a common mistake is to enter blood pressure as 120/80. Those data should be stored as two columns, with one holding systolic pressure, and the other holding diastolic pressure; otherwise, it is extremely difficult to calculate the average systolic pressure. Another common mistake is to include the units of measurement in the column (e.g. enter '10 days old' or '1 month of age' in the spreadsheet cells). Instead, the variable should allow only one type of data (e.g. days), and values should be entered with only the analysable number (e.g. 10 or 30).

Spreadsheets like Microsoft Excel allow any value to be typed into any cell. This is potentially dangerous because it allows a researcher to enter 'blue' into the age column or to make even more pernicious mistakes like entering a lab value as <1.0 to indicate the floor value from a lab assay. Entering < or > symbols causes the cell to be treated as character data, and this can cause Excel to exclude that value when the data is exported for analysis. Columns in Excel can be set to 'validate' values and give the user clues to the possible values. That is, when a user selects a cell it shows permitted values and blocks invalid data entry (such as a 'green' gender, or dates before the start of the study).

Most software packages will not accept variable names that are 30 or more characters long and, even if accepted, may abbreviate for display purposes, so use short but descriptive names. Spaces within variable names are not generally allowed in software packages even though they are allowed in spreadsheets. Words can be separated with an underscore '_' character, as in date_of_death, or compressed with each word beginning with a capital letter, as in DateOfDeath. The first character of the name should be a letter, not a number, although numbers can go anywhere else (e.g. 'pulse1'). Repeat measures should be given similar but unique names (e.g. 'diast1' and 'diast2' for the first and second diastolic blood pressure values, respectively). As mentioned in subsection 2.4.3, a record of the meaning of the variable names should be kept with the coding schedule/data dictionary. If you are asking yes/no questions, it can be helpful to include a leading verb in the variable name—e.g. the variable 'isMale' coded with 1 = Yes, 0 = No, is easily interpretable compared to 'gender' 1 = Female vs. 2 = Male.

Note that in figure 2.1 there are no gaps in the rows and columns, and only one row is used for the variable names. Where the subjects are in several groups all data should be in one spreadsheet, rather than in several, with the group identity indicated by a group variable in a separate column. If data are entered or stored in this format they will be much easier to transfer into a statistical package.

Data collection forms can be designed with specialized software, such as TeleForm (http://www.electricpaper.biz/products/teleform.html), so that they can be scanned directly into the computer when completed (see figure 2.2). This may save time but is not entirely trouble-free as the scanner may misread data if responses are slightly out of alignment, or the handwriting is unclear. Tick boxes usually scan correctly but handwritten numbers may not; for example, badly written 7s can look like 9s and lead to scanning errors. Hence, some checking is still needed when scanning is used.

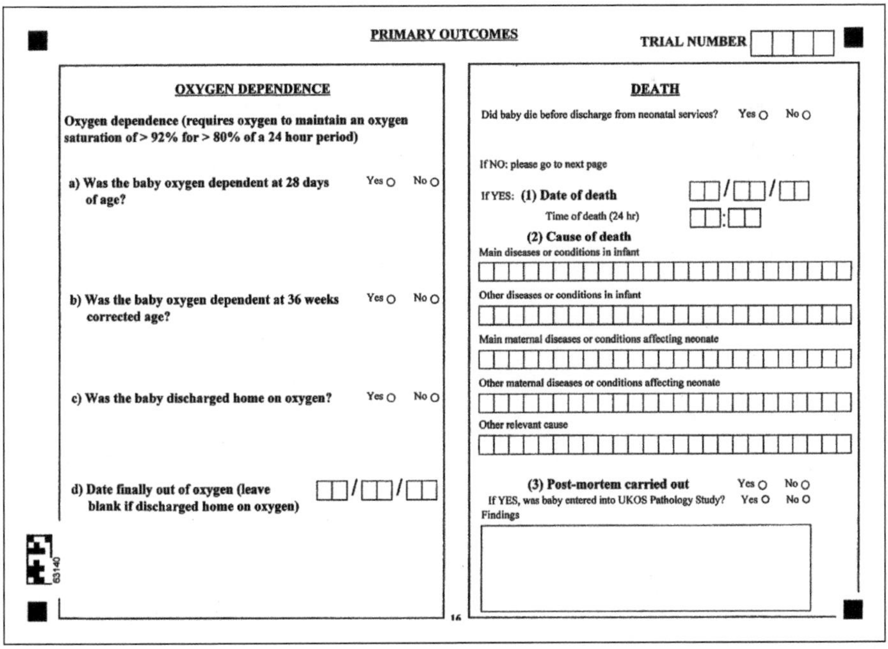
PRIMARY OUTCOMES

TRIAL NUMBER

OXYGEN DEPENDENCE

Oxygen dependence (requires oxygen to maintain an oxygen saturation of > 92% for > 80% of a 24 hour period)

a) Was the baby oxygen dependent at 28 days of age? Yes ○ No ○

b) Was the baby oxygen dependent at 36 weeks corrected age? Yes ○ No ○

c) Was the baby discharged home on oxygen? Yes ○ No ○

d) Date finally out of oxygen (leave blank if discharged home on oxygen) __/__/__

DEATH

Did baby die before discharge from neonatal services? Yes ○ No ○

If NO: please go to next page

If YES: (1) Date of death __/__/__

Time of death (24 hr) __:__

(2) Cause of death

Main diseases or conditions in infant

Other diseases or conditions in infant

Main maternal diseases or conditions affecting neonate

Other maternal diseases or conditions affecting neonate

Other relevant cause

(3) Post-mortem carried out Yes ○ No ○

If YES, was baby entered into UKOS Pathology Study? Yes ○ No ○

Findings

63140

16

Figure 2.2 Example of a form that can be scanned

2.5 Data checking and cleaning

It is advisable to check the data as the study progresses rather than leave it until the end, as early checks may reveal problems that can be resolved. The process of data checking and cleaning involves looking for unlikely or impossible values or outliers; for example, 'diast2=182'—a very high value for diastolic blood pressure—should be checked (figure 2.3). Possible errors like this can be identified if summary statistics and/or a histogram of the data are produced (figure 2.4). In some data-entry programs, including REDCap, the user can set acceptable limits for each variable and thus force the computer to flag or reject values outside that range. If there is no evidence of a mistake, and the value is plausible, then it should not be altered. It is good practice to keep a record of all checks that have been made, and the results of the decisions, including the date and initials of the person making each decision, even if the data are not changed. For a fuller discussion of outliers see Altman 1991 (chapter 7).

Errors can also occur where the data have been incorrectly entered but the value entered is a possible value and so is not flagged. This sort of error is very difficult to detect. Entering the data twice, 'double entry', can minimize errors although errors due to ambiguity in handwriting may be entered wrongly twice. To look for these sorts of mistakes it can be useful to hand-check a sample of forms to estimate the extent of any problems. If problems appear to be present then further hand-checking, particularly for key variables, is advisable. This is another reason why it is a good idea to do some quality checks early on in the study.

Data inconsistent: Patient does not have rhinitis but answered question about when rhinitis occurred

Value outside likely range: Diastolic blood pressure high although possible. However, measurements also inconsistent with first and second readings; possible transcription error?

patid	age	yob	rhinitis	whenrh	pulse1	syst1	diast1	pulse2	syst2	diast2	pulse3	syst3	diast3
1	72	1929	0	4	51	164	72	53	152	126	55	157	71
2	46	1955	0	4	86	159	90	84	153	98	84	125	82
3	80		0	4	111	130	63	33	211	182	111	109	60
4	70	1931	0	4	65	102	55	68	95	59	74	97	56
5	62	1939	0	1	97	141	85	94	141	84	101	143	82
6	75	1926	0	4	63	161	100	62	153	90	62	156	89
7	47	1954	0	4	80	123	67	82	101	65	81	101	66
8	72		0	4	88	169	89	88	151	94	87	156	76
9	63	1938	0	4	64	129	85	68	142	84	64	142	84
10	85	1926	1	3	71	97	62	67	98	54	71	94	56
11	42	1958	0	4	78	112	71	70	108	68	74	109	68
12	75	1926	1	3	98	157	87	95	149	83	98	138	78
13	68	1933	1	3	105	134	73	103	130	65	103	116	60
14	40		0	4	91	122	74	85	109	79	97	111	74

Inconsistent data: Person born in 1926 would be 75 in 2001 when study carried out

Value outside likely range: Diastolic blood pressure and systolic blood pressure too high and pulse too low. Measurements also inconsistent with first and second readings; likely that machine was not working properly for this set of readings.

Figure 2.3 Checking for errors in the data (example)

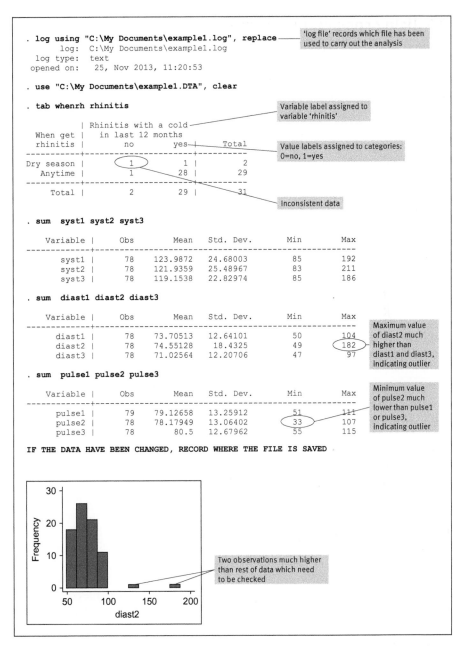

Figure 2.4 Output to check data and to show the use of a 'log' file to record the results of the analysis (Stata)

Another type of data error is internal inconsistency, for example 'rhinitis=0' ('no rhinitis') and 'whenrhin=1' ('have rhinitis in the dry season'). This was noticed when the data were cross-tabulated. In some cases it may not be obvious which responses are correct. Where there is doubt, it is advisable to discuss the options with another team member and/or the statistician who will analyse the data.

2.6 Using computer packages

There are many commercially produced statistical packages available, such as SAS, R, Stata, SPSS, JMP, S-Plus, Minitab, and countless more. The choice of which to use will depend on your budget, on ease of access to support staff, on what analyses you want to do, and to some extent on your personal preferences. There are also other public domain statistical programs and spreadsheets that are available free or at minimal cost (box 2.9). Some of these will calculate confidence intervals from summary data. This may be particularly useful for SPSS users since SPSS does not always give confidence intervals.

In this book we demonstrate the use of SAS, R, Stata, and SPSS for statistical analyses and, in addition, we use Epi-Info and G*Power for sample size calculations. Boxes 2.9 and 2.10 list the main features of each of these and a few other selected programs, and box 2.11 gives some books that we have found useful.

Menu-driven programs provide the user with a list of possibilities to choose from. Many users like selecting from menus since it does not require them to learn the syntax of commands. The disadvantages of menu-driven programs include their inflexibility, their relative slowness if a complex procedure is required, and the difficulty of remembering how to repeat a complex analysis. Ideally, users can point-and-click their way to an analysis and then study the code to learn how to quickly and easily expand the analysis. Command-driven programs require the user to write commands according to a specific, often arcane, syntax in order to carry out the analysis. If the syntax is even slightly wrongly typed, the command will not execute.

Spreadsheets are useful for entering and manipulating data, and some researchers use them for data analysis. In general we are cautious about recommending this since the scope of the analyses tends to be limited, unless specialized modules are added on.

It is good practice at the outset of a study to write a statistical analysis plan (SAP) to guide the analysis (see section 2.7). In particular, randomized controlled trials require an SAP to be written and logged prior to any data analyses, including analyses for data monitoring purposes. This will ensure that the analyses performed answer the original study questions and prevent ad hoc analyses and spurious significant findings.

SAS, R, Stata, and SPSS produce detailed results for many analyses, and not all of these are appropriate to all situations. This book shows examples of many analyses and indicates which results apply in particular situations, but researchers are advised to be careful and to read the user manual if in any doubt, or to seek advice from an experienced user. It is important to check the assumptions underlying any statistical procedures and only to report the results which you understand. If the assumptions which the analysis makes about the data are not true, then results may be invalid. Unfortunately, the computer may not warn you about this, so it is all too easy to produce analyses which look fine but are in fact meaningless.

2.7 Record keeping

Good record keeping is an essential part of the statistical analysis. You should be able to know who did what to the data, and when, throughout the life of your project, and records should be kept of data coding, checking, cleaning, and analysis, and the results (box 2.12). This audit trail is mandatory for submissions to regulatory agencies in the United States

**Box 2.9 Some software available on the www, free or
at modest price**   *INFORMATION*

Epi-Info (http://www.cdc.gov/epiinfo)
- Written primarily for case-control studies but can be used with other designs
- Menu- or command-driven
- Will be used in this book for sample size calculations for proportions
- Also performs basic statistical analyses (not covered here)

G*Power (http://www.psycho.uni-duesseldorf.de/abteilungen/aap/
gpower3)
- Full-featured power and sample size calculator
- Free

Clinstat (http://www-users.york.ac.uk/~mb55/)
- Written by Martin Bland, York University, UK
- DOS-based menu-driven program
- Basic statistical analysis from data or summary statistics
- Sample size calculations

Biconf (http://www-users.york.ac.uk/~mb55/)
- Written by Martin Bland, York University, UK
- Exact confidence intervals for rates and proportions

CIPROPORTION and other spreadsheet calculators (https://www.crcpress.
com/Confidence-Intervals-for-Proportions-and-Related-Measures-of-Effect-
Size/Newcombe/p/book/9781439812785)
- Written by Robert Newcombe, Cardiff University, UK
- Annotated Excel spreadsheets—the user enters their summary data
- Easy to use

Confidence Interval analysis (http:/www.som.soton.ac.uk/cia/)
- Accompanies the book *Statistics with Confidence* (Altman et al. 2000)
- Book purchase required for license key

Stats Direct (http://www.statsdirect.com)
- Written for medical researchers
- Wide range of statistical analyses applicable to medicine
- Easy to use
- Emphasis on confidence intervals
- 10-day free trial

Box 2.10 Commercial programs illustrated in this book	*INFORMATION*

SAS

- Not for Mac OS
- Widely used by statisticians and some medical researchers
- Command driven
- Moderately complex command structure
- Simple to complex analysis
- Excellent connectivity with databases
- Excellent technical support, books, and manuals
- Sample size calculations for many designs
- Cost prohibitive outside of academic use

SAS University Edition

- Mac, Windows, and others
- Used by medical researchers
- Point-and-click and command driven
- Writes some SAS commands for you
- Simple to complex analysis
- Sample size calculations for many designs
- Free for academic use

R

- Mac, Windows and others
- Widely used by statisticians
- Easy to very difficult command structure
- Simple to very complex analysis
- Fair to good connectivity with databases
- Very poor help files, no commercial tech support, but many web resources/ book refs
- Sample size calculations for many designs
- Free

Stata

- Mac, Windows, and others
- Widely used by statisticians and medical researchers
- Command driven and menu driven, Windows based
- Simple command structure
- Simple to complex analysis
- Excellent help files
- Sample size calculations for proportions and means
- Cost: varying tiers depending on user status and size of package

Box 2.10 *continued*

SPSS

- Mac, Windows, and others
- Widely used by social scientists and medical researchers
- Menu driven, Windows based
- Can run from commands but syntax is relatively complicated
- Simple to complex analysis
- Does not do sample size calculations
- Cost: varying tiers depending on user status and packages purchased

Box 2.11 Some useful books on statistical packages   *INFORMATION*

Here we list just a few books that we have found helpful. We know there are many, many more out there. We suggest that you look at any book before buying to see if it meets your needs, as they vary enormously in scope and detail.

SAS

- Ron Cody. *Learning SAS by Example: A Programmer's Guide*. SAS Institute 2007.
- Glenn Walker, Jack Shostak. *Common Statistical Methods for Clinical Research with SAS Examples*, Third Edition. SAS Institute 2010.
- Paul D. Allison. *Survival Analysis Using SAS: A Practical Guide*, Second Edition. SAS Institute 2010.
- Paul D. Allison. *Logistic Regression Using SAS: Theory and Application*, Second Edition. SAS Institute 2012.

Stata

- Brian S. Everitt and Sophia Rabe-Hesketh. *Handbook of Statistical Analyses Using Stata*, Fourth Edition. Chapman and Hall 2006

SPSS

- Louise Marston. *Introductory Statistics for Health and Nursing Using SPSS*. Sage Publications 2009.

R

- Alain F. Zuur, Elena N. Ieno, Erik Meesters. *A Beginner's Guide to R (Use R!)*. Springer 2009.
- Robert Kabacoff. *R in Action: Data Analysis and Graphics with R*. Manning Publications 2015.
- John Maindonald and W. John Braun. *Data Analysis and Graphics Using R: An Example-Based Approach*. Cambridge University Press 2010.

Box 2.12 Good record keeping   *HELPFUL TIPS*

- Use a data dictionary (written coding schedule; see table 2.1) and record any amendments clearly and systematically along with the date and the initials of the person making the change
- Record all checks which have been carried out, including those where data are unchanged, e.g. *'unusual value; checked against questionnaire and no errors found'*
- Record any changes made to individual participant data with an explanation if necessary, e.g. *'impossible value, set to missing'*
- Use a computer log file to record any changes made to the data on the computer (see figure 2.4)
- Use a computer log file as in figure 2.4 to record the results of the analysis and commands used to produce the results

Remember, others may need to check or use your data, or check your research results at a later stage.

---

and Europe but should be considered standard practice regardless of your legal responsibilities. Most programs will produce an electronic copy or log file of the results of the analyses, which will record the names of the data files used and the commands that have been run to make any changes to the data, and to carry out the statistical analysis. An example using Stata is shown in figure 2.4. Having a log file means that any analysis can easily be reproduced. This will save a lot of time if the analysis needs to be repeated, for example, if an error is discovered in the data. Only the parts of the log file relevant to the analysis being demonstrated will be shown in the rest of this book.

2.8 Presenting results

When we present results, either orally or in writing, we want our audience or readers to be interested in, and to understand, the message we are giving. If the presentation is unclear or muddled, or just too long, then the attention of the audience or readers may be lost; hence the need to present results in a clear and logical way that clearly communicates the findings.

The format of the presentation will depend on the medium—written or oral; for example, a graph or chart may be used to show results in an oral presentation, while a table would be used in a written document. These aspects will be addressed in detail in chapter 5.

2.9 When to seek help from a statistician

We advise researchers to consult a medical statistician early in the protocol development phase.

A medical statistician is able to help with design issues as well as perform sample size calculations and do chi-squared tests! Some studies which appear to be straightforward may involve subtle design or analysis issues. This is particularly true of randomized controlled trials which need to be rigorously carried out, so advice on design and analysis is best obtained at the planning stage.

Other things that statisticians can advise on include questionnaire design, planning the analysis (to be done at the outset), writing up in general, and interpreting the results. If the study is complex, such as a large cohort study or a multi-centre clinical trial, then the research team should include a statistician to take part in actually running the study as well as taking responsibility for analysing the data, and grant bids should include realistic costs for the statistician's time.

Box 2.13 Key points when planning research   *CHAPTER SUMMARY*

- Define a research question that can be answered
- Write a protocol at the outset
- Seek statistical advice early on
- Only collect data you really need
- Enter data onto a computer in an appropriate format
- Check data quality early on
- Consider involving a statistician as a collaborator

CHAPTER 3

Writing a research protocol

3.1 **The development cycle** *22*

3.2 **Title** *22*

3.3 **Aims of the research study** *23*

3.4 **Primary and secondary aims** *24*

3.5 **Study design** *24*

3.6 **Sample size calculations** *24*

3.7 **Plan of statistical analysis** *34*

3.8 **Required approval for research** *34*

3.9 **When applications fail** *38*

3.1 The development cycle

A good research protocol describes the details of, and the rationale for, the research study that is being proposed. This is not to be confused with a clinical treatment protocol (box 3.1), which describes how patients should be managed. The main components of a research protocol are described in chapter 2 (box 2.4). This chapter deals with the sample size calculations and plan of statistical analysis in more detail. However, these aspects cannot be considered in isolation; developing a protocol is often an iterative process, as initial ideas are thought through, problems identified, the question redefined, and so on. For example, a researcher may have a good idea, a sound study design, and a robust outcome measure, but having calculated the required sample size he finds that the proposed study cannot be achieved in the available time, and/or with the available resources. Alternatively, background reading may reveal that the chosen research question has already been answered, or that a proposed intervention is unlikely to have the desired effect (box 3.2). It is far better to identify such problems at the outset than later on when trying to get the study published.

3.2 Title

The project should be given a title that clearly reflects the aims of the study. The title introduces the readers to the project and is the first indication the reader has about what the researcher is trying to do. Careful thought needs to be given to the title so that it is accurate, not too long, and intelligible to the non-specialist. Sometimes, the title is included on a patient information sheet, in which case it will need to be written in relatively simple language.

Box 3.1 How a research protocol differs from other protocols   *INFORMATION*

Research protocol

- Why the study is being carried out
- What is to be done and by whom
- How the results are going to be analysed

Clinical protocol

- Clinical protocols or guidelines are used to determine good practice in different clinical situations, e.g. how patients should be managed
- May be part of a *research* protocol but is not sufficient in itself for a research study

Standard Operating Procedures (SOPs)

- For larger studies it may be advisable to write a fuller protocol after funding has been agreed. This may be accompanied by a set of Standard Operating Procedures which describe what to do in specific situations.

3.3 Aims of the research study

A research protocol is analogous to a route planning map. We need to know where we are going (the aims) and have a broad view of how we are going to get there (the study design) but also include some finer details so we know what to do at certain points on the journey (details such as recruitment procedures). We also need to justify why we are going there,

---

Box 3.2 Redefining a research aim   *EXAMPLE*

Aim 1

- *To reduce the number of miscarriages due to infection*

This is not a research aim. It is doing something to improve health rather than finding something out.

Aim 2

- *To investigate whether screening and treating women for bacterial vaginosis reduces the chance of early miscarriage*

This asks a question but may not be achievable since it would require a large, and therefore expensive, randomized controlled trial screening some women and not others. This would only be justified if there was sufficient evidence that bacterial vaginosis is associated with early miscarriage.

Aim 3

- To determine if bacterial vaginosis detected before 10 weeks is associated with miscarriage before 16 weeks

This aim answers a question, is achievable within the funding constraints and is appropriate to current knowledge.

especially if other people may be inconvenienced in the process (background). Unless we are clear about where we are going we cannot plan an efficient route. Similarly, without clear aims it is impossible to write a good research protocol.

Research is about finding out and asking questions. Research aims should clearly state what the project is aiming to find out. While the motive for research may be to improve the care of patients, and this may be a worthwhile aim, it is not a research aim. This is illustrated in the example in box 3.2. A clear statement of aims makes writing, reading, and reviewing a protocol much easier.

3.4 Primary and secondary aims

Sometimes researchers may want to answer several questions from one study. This is often because collecting the data is time-consuming and expensive and so the researchers want to make the best use of the data. However, there are drawbacks. If too many hypotheses are tested in a study then there is an increased chance of spurious statistical significance. For a fuller discussion of this see Bland 2015 (chapter 9). Altman 1991 (chapter 15) recommends that trials should have only one primary outcome, and that other outcomes should be considered to be of secondary importance. This is illustrated by the UKOS trial (box 3.3).

3.5 Study design

Box 3.4 outlines the main issues that need to be clarified when writing the study design section. This can then form the basis of the methods section when writing up the study.

3.6 Sample size calculations

At the outset of a study a decision has to be made as to how many subjects are going to be recruited. The study can then be costed and its feasibility assessed. The number should be large enough to avoid inconclusive results and yet not so large that subjects are put to unnecessary inconvenience and the study becomes unnecessarily expensive.

Box 3.3 Primary and secondary aims—UKOS study   *EXAMPLE*

Primary aim

Does early intervention with high-frequency oscillatory ventilation reduce mortality and incidence of chronic lung disease among babies with gestational age <29 weeks, compared with conventional ventilation?

Secondary aim

Does high-frequency oscillatory ventilation affect age at death, age at discharge, major cranial abnormality, air leak, failure of treatment, hearing, necrotizing enterocolitis, patent ductus arteriosus, postnatal systemic steroid use, pulmonary haemorrhage, and retinopathy of prematurity?

Study design

Randomized controlled trial

| Box 3.4 Writing a protocol—study design | *INFORMATION* |

Type of study; most studies will be one of the following

- Intervention study (trial)—randomized or not
- Cohort study
- Cross-sectional survey
- Case-control study

Discuss reason for choice of design and its advantages and disadvantages.

Selection of subjects

- Define population.
- How will subjects be selected? What sampling method will be used?
- Describe and justify recruitment procedures (are they feasible?).
- What steps will be taken to ensure a high response rate?
- How many subjects will be required and how was this chosen?
- State inclusion and exclusion criteria.

Data collection and analysis

- What data are to be collected and why?
- What factors are thought to affect the outcome?
- What factors may distort the representativeness of the findings?
- What are the outcome measures in the study?
- Is it possible to collect these data?

How will the data be collected and by whom?

- Questionnaires, interviews, or routine data sources?
- Have any questionnaires proposed been validated?
- Will staff training be required?
- What measures are taken to avoid bias (e.g. blinding among patients, assessors, and data analysts)?

How will the data be processed?

- On a computer database?
- Will the data be validated?
- What steps have been taken to ensure data confidentiality?

There are various sources of information available which describe how to do basic sample size calculations and give explanations of the terms involved (Peacock and Peacock 2011 (chapter 1), Altman 1991, Bland 2015, http://www-users.york.ac.uk/~mb55/guide/guide.htm). The actual sample size calculations may be carried out by hand, using either a calculator or a diagram called a nomogram (Altman 1991, Petrie and Sabin 2009), using books of tables (Machin et al. 2008), or using a statistics package (e.g. G*Power, Epi-Info (table 2.1), Stata, NQuery, PASS).

The presentation of the results of such calculations in the protocol, with reference to output from G*Power, Stata, and Epi-Info in the three most common scenarios (prevalence studies, studies comparing two proportions, and studies comparing two means), is described in this chapter.

3.6.1 Prevalence studies

These involve the study of one group of people in order to estimate the prevalence of a disease in that group. No comparisons are being made and no significance tests are carried out but the precision of our estimate of prevalence can be specified by calculating the confidence interval, usually the 95% confidence interval. This is a range of values which has a 95% probability of containing the true population prevalence we are trying to estimate.

Box 3.5 lists the information required to do the calculations, which can be done in Epi-Info. Box 3.6 gives an example of a sample size statement from a survey of women to estimate the prevalence of chlamydia infection. All the assumptions made are contained in the sample size statement, and prior information is referenced. Figure 3.1 shows the output from Epi-Info related to this calculation. The number of subjects was rounded up from 1276 to 1300 in the protocol.

3.6.2 Screening studies (sensitivity and specificity)

Studies to estimate sensitivity and specificity are also based on proportions but have the added complication that each proportion will be calculated using only part of the sample. The number of subjects for the sensitivity calculation is the number of true positives, and the number of subjects for the specificity is the number of true negatives. If the expected number of true positives is low, then even if the total sample is large the estimate of the sensitivity may be imprecise and thus have a wide confidence interval.

Where the true status of the patients is not known in advance, the prevalence will also need to be estimated. This is illustrated by a cohort study to test a non-invasive antenatal screening method for chromosomal abnormalities (box 3.7). The true status of the baby may not be known until birth and so all babies would need to be screened and followed up to see which of those that test positive were really affected. The prevalence

---

Box 3.5 Information required for sample size calculations for estimating a prevalence with a certain accuracy　　*INFORMATION*

An estimate of the size of prevalence expected This can be obtained from pilot studies or published studies. If there is no information available use 0.50 or 50%, which will tend to be conservative, i.e. overestimate the sample size.

Confidence level This is usually set to 95% but can be 90% or 99%.

Required width of the confidence interval The researcher decides how precise the estimate is to be and this determines how wide the interval must be. The accuracy will usually be half the width of the interval; e.g. in estimating a proportion expected to be close to 40%, the researcher may decide that this should be accurate to within 2 percentage points, i.e. ±2 percentage points. Thus, the width of the confidence interval will be 4 percentage points.

Box 3.6 Sample size statement for chlamydia prevalence study *EXAMPLE*

Chlamydia study

Aim

To calculate the prevalence of chlamydia infection among women attending primary care for cervical smears

Information required

- Estimate of the prevalence = 7% (from previous studies)
- Confidence level = 95% (decided by the researcher)
- Accuracy of ±1.4 percentage points (decided by the researcher)

Required sample size

1300 women (from Epi-Info)

Sample size statement

'1300 women would allow estimation of the prevalence of chlamydia infection to within 1.4 percentage points either side of the estimated prevalence, using a 95% confidence interval, assuming that the prevalence is approximately 7%'

The estimate of prevalence came from unpublished data from another researcher.

For further information see Oakeshott P, Kerry S, H S, Hay P. Opportunistic screening for chlamydial infection at time of cervical smear testing in general practice: prevalence study. *BMJ* 1998; 316:351–352.

---

of chromosomal abnormalities is very low so even with a large sample there will be few babies who are true positives from which to estimate the sensitivity. It may be that we have to accept wide confidence intervals, but it is useful to know the limitations of the study in advance.

3.6.3 Comparison studies

These involve comparing two or more groups of subjects, and the outcome might be either a proportion or a mean. Consideration needs to be given to what kind of difference is of such clinical importance that the study will be statistically significant if this difference really exists in the whole population. The information required in order to carry out the calculation is given in boxes 3.8 and 3.10.

3.6.4 Computer packages

G*Power and Stata will estimate sample sizes for either a difference of means or a difference of proportions; Epi-Info will only compare percentages (proportions). Examples of output are given in figures 3.1 to 3.3. Stata expresses power and significance levels as proportions, but power is normally expressed as a percentage in sample size statements. Epi-Info expresses significance as the confidence level, which is 100-significance. So if the required significance level is 5%, then 95% is entered into the 'confidence' box in Epi-Info. PASS and nQuery Advisor will do simple and more complex sample size calculations, but they need to be purchased.

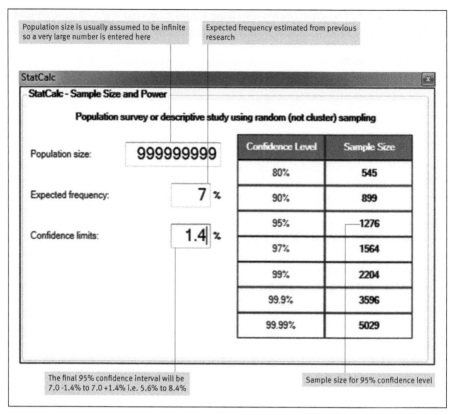

Population size is usually assumed to be infinite so a very large number is entered here

Expected frequency estimated from previous research

StatCalc

StatCalc - Sample Size and Power

Population survey or descriptive study using random (not cluster) sampling

Population size: 999999999

Expected frequency: 7 %

Confidence limits: 1.4 %

Confidence Level	Sample Size
80%	545
90%	899
95%	1276
97%	1564
99%	2204
99.9%	3596
99.99%	5029

The final 95% confidence interval will be 7.0 -1.4% to 7.0 +1.4% i.e. 5.6% to 8.4%

Sample size for 95% confidence level

Figure 3.1 Output for sample size for a prevalence (Epi-Info)

3.6.5 Sample size for two proportions

The power is related to the minimum difference between the two proportions, expressed as a risk difference, relative risk, or odds ratio. G*Power requires the user to specify the two proportions which make up that difference, not the difference. Epi-Info is more flexible and requires one percentage and then either the second percentage or the relative risk or the odds ratio.

Box 3.8 summarizes the information required to carry out a sample size calculation for comparing two proportions. Box 3.9 shows an example of a sample size statement to compare two proportions taken from a randomized controlled trial comparing two methods of ventilation in babies (UKOS study). The calculations are shown in figure 3.2.

3.6.6 Sample size for two means

Box 3.10 shows the information required to carry out a sample size calculation to compare two means—instead of an estimate of the prevalence in one group, an estimate of the standard deviation is needed. The calculations can be done in Stata or G*Power but not in Epi-Info. When calculating sample sizes for the difference between two means, G*Power requires either both means and standard deviation to be given, or the effect size (difference in means divided by the standard deviation) (figure 3.3). In practice the absolute value of the means does not matter, only the difference between them—for example, with the

Box 3.7 Sample size for sensitivity	*EXAMPLE*

Aim

To calculate the sensitivity and specificity of nuchal translucency screening for chromosomal abnormalities using an unselected cohort of pregnant women

Information required

- Estimate of the prevalence of chromosomal abnormalities = 1% (from previous studies)
- Estimate of sensitivity (from previous studies) = 70%
- Confidence level = 95% (decided by the researcher)
- Accuracy of ±20 percentage points (decided by the researcher)

Required sample size

20 babies with chromosomal abnormalities (1% or 0.01 of population) and hence 2000 pregnant women required overall (20/0.01 = 2000)

Sample size statement

'2000 pregnant women are likely to have 20 babies with chromosomal abnormalities. This would allow the sensitivity of the test to be estimated to within ±20 percentage points using a 95% confidence interval, assuming that the sensitivity is approximately 70%'

birthweight data, the same sample size would be obtained if the two means were 2000 and 2180. This principle does not hold for proportions where the sample size depends not only on the difference but also on the absolute value of the proportions.

Box 3.11 gives an example of a sample size statement from a study comparing mean birthweight in two groups. The output for G*Power is given in figure 3.3. Note that, in this

Box 3.8 Information required to compare two proportions	*INFORMATION*

Estimate of proportion in one group Can be obtained from pilot studies, other publications

Significance level Usually set to 5%, but sometimes 1% or lower

Power The probability of detecting a specified size of effect if it exists. Power usually set to 80% or 90%.

The smallest effect of interest This needs to be decided by the researcher. It is the size of effect that is clinically important. This may be a difference of proportions (risk difference), relative risk, or odds ratio.

The ratio of the numbers of subjects in each group For most randomized trials this will be 1, i.e. the groups will all be the same size but group sizes may be very different in observational studies (e.g. comparing smokers and non-smokers where there are more non-smokers in the population than smokers).

Box 3.9 Sample size statement for comparing two proportions   *EXAMPLE*

United Kingdom Oscillation Study (UKOS)
Aim

To compare prevalence of death or chronic lung disease in premature babies randomized to two methods of ventilation

Outcome

Death or chronic lung disease at 36 weeks postmenstrual age

Information required

◆ Estimate of the prevalence in control group = 67% (from previous studies)
◆ Significance level = 5% (decided by the researcher)
◆ Risk difference to be detected 11 percentage points (i.e.to 56% in intervention group, decided by the researcher)
◆ Power 90% (decided by researcher)
◆ Babies will be randomized to two equal-sized groups

Required sample size

428 babies in each group (from Stata)

Sample size statement

428 babies in each group would allow a difference of 11 percentage points in the prevalence of death or chronic lung disease at 36 weeks post menstrual age, assuming that the prevalence is 56% in the control group with a power of 90%, using a 5% significance level

Note: This example has been simplified here for illustration. The UKOS study actually considered a range of possible sample sizes from 800– to 1200 since it was uncertain at the outset how many babies could be recruited in the time available. The paper reports this in detail and also gives a full justification of the control group prevalence (see chapter 10 for details).

For further information see Johnson AH, Peacock JL, Greenough A, Marlow N, Limb ES, Marston L et al. High-frequency oscillatory ventilation for the prevention of chronic lung disease of prematurity. *N Engl J Med* 2002; 347:633–642.

example, the calculated sample size was inflated because the study was aimed at detecting differences between social class subgroups which were only 10% of the total sample. Hence, if the 10% subgroup needed to contain 164 subjects, then the total sample size needed to be 1630.

3.6.7 Unequal sized groups

In most randomized controlled trials the treatment groups are equal in size because this is the most efficient design. However, this is not always possible. If the ratio of subjects in one group to the other is not equal, i.e. not 1.0, then the sample size calculations can still be done by specifying this ratio. In Stata this is done by adding an extra command to the

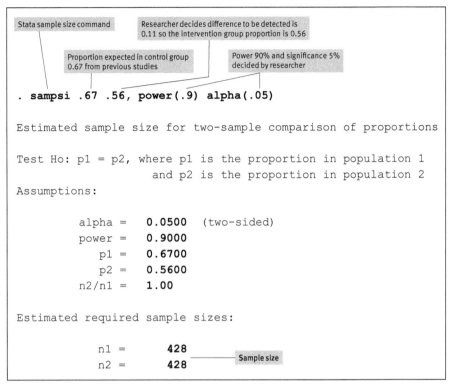

```
. sampsi .67 .56, power(.9) alpha(.05)

Estimated sample size for two-sample comparison of proportions

Test Ho: p1 = p2, where p1 is the proportion in population 1
                   and p2 is the proportion in population 2
Assumptions:

             alpha =   0.0500   (two-sided)
             power =   0.9000
                p1 =   0.6700
                p2 =   0.5600
             n2/n1 =   1.00

Estimated required sample sizes:

                n1 =      428
                n2 =      428
```

Figure 3.2 Output for sample size for two proportions (Stata)

sampsi statement. So, if the required ratio of sample sizes, n_2/n_1, was 2, then **r(2)** would be added to the command line after the comma (see figure 3.2). Epi- Info and G*Power also allow calculations with unequal sample sizes.

If we do not know how many subjects fall into each group, it is useful to carry out a sensitivity analysis on the sample size calculations and to recalculate the sample size using different assumptions.

Box 3.10 Information required to compare two means   *INFORMATION*

Estimate of standard deviation Can be obtained from pilot studies, other publications

Significance level Usually set to 5%, but sometimes 1% or lower

Power The probability of detecting a specified size of effect if it exists. Usually set to 80% or 90%

The smallest effect of interest This is the difference between the groups that is clinically important. The researcher needs to decide this.

The ratio of the numbers of subjects in each group For most randomized trials this will be 1, i.e. the groups will all be the same size but group sizes may be very different in observational studies.

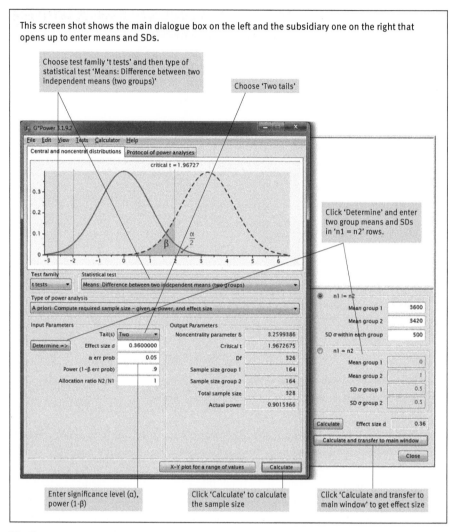

This screen shot shows the main dialogue box on the left and the subsidiary one on the right that opens up to enter means and SDs.

Choose test family 't tests' and then type of statistical test 'Means: Difference between two independent means (two groups)'

Choose 'Two tails'

Click 'Determine' and enter two group means and SDs in 'n1 = n2' rows.

Enter significance level (α), power (1-β)

Click 'Calculate' to calculate the sample size

Click 'Calculate and transfer to main window' to get effect size

📑 **Figure 3.3** Output for sample size of the difference between two means (G*Power)

3.6.8 Subgroup and multifactorial analyses

Stata 13 and G*Power plus commercial packages will do sample size calculations for some more complex analyses such as analysis of variance and some multifactorial regressions, but these require the user to provide more prior information than simple analyses and so are not straightforward to use. We suggest that statistical advice is sought if such analyses are planned.

3.6.9 Cluster randomized trials

Most drug trials randomize individual participants to treatment groups. However, for trials investigating the effectiveness of different methods of health service delivery, whole groups (clusters) of individuals may be randomized. These are commonly known as cluster randomized trials and, in the UK, general practices are often randomized as a cluster. If

---

Box 3.11 Sample size statement for comparing two means   *EXAMPLE*

Birthweight study

Aim
To compare mean birthweight of babies in different social class subgroups

Outcome
Birthweight

Information required
◆ Estimate of the standard deviation of birthweight = 500 g (from previous studies)
◆ Significance level = 5% (decided by the researcher)
◆ Difference to be detected 180 g (decided by researcher)
◆ Power 90% (decided by researcher)

Required sample size
164 women in each group

Sample size statement
The target sample size was 328. This sample size is sufficient to detect differences in mean birthweight between two social class subgroups, with power 90%. A 5% (two-sided) significance level was assumed and a standard deviation of 500 g.

Note: The study wanted to be able to detect differences in subgroups as small as 10% of the total sample and so the target sample size was multiplied by 10 to give a final target sample of 1630 women.

For further information see Brooke OG, Anderson HR, Bland JM, Peacock JL, Stewart CM. Effects on birth weight of smoking, alcohol, caffeine, socioeconomic factors, and psychosocial stress. *BMJ* 1989; 298:795–801.

---

the clustering is ignored when the sample size calculations are done, the resultant number will be an underestimate of the true sample size required, and in some cases the underestimation is substantial. Methods to calculate sample size for cluster trials are described in Eldridge and Kerry 2012, Kerry and Bland 1998a, and Donner and Klar 2000.

3.6.10 Presentation of sample size statements

Examples of sample size statements are given in boxes 3.6, 3.7, 3.9, and 3.11. Where results from other studies have been used, these should be referenced and any assumptions made should be clearly stated. It is important to state not only the power, and the significance level, but also the difference to be detected. This is because, as the difference to be detected increases, so does the power of the study for the same level of significance. Because virtually all tests should be two-sided this is not always stated explicitly, although there is no harm in doing so for complete clarity (box 3.11).

In box 3.9 the sample size statement expresses the difference between the two percentages as '11 percentage points' difference rather than 11 per cent, to avoid confusion. An 11% difference would imply 56% in one group and 62% in the other ($1.11 \times 0.56 \times 100$).

3.6.11 Feasibility

Along with the sample size statements, it is useful to give evidence of the feasibility of the planned sample size, particularly in grant applications. For example, in the UKOS study, the number of eligible babies normally admitted to a unit in a year was presented in the application and protocol to show that the target recruitment was feasible. For some studies it is not clear if the target recruitment is feasible and so a prior, small-scale feasibility study may be needed to check this out.

3.7 Plan of statistical analysis

A plan of statistical analysis should be presented in the protocol and there are several reasons for preparing this plan in advance. First, it identifies any problems with the analysis that might indicate that a different study design would be better. Second, stating the main analysis in advance demonstrates that it was pre-planned. This protects against the possibility of the researcher changing the main outcome or method of analysis if the first outcome or method does not give the anticipated or desired results, thus giving the results more credibility and ensuring that the study is fairly reported. Carrying out 100 different analyses and only reporting those which show significant findings gives a biased view of the results of the study. If the original research question is interesting and useful then the results will be worth presenting regardless of whether they are statistically significant or not, provided the study has been properly carried out. What is of less interest is a poorly conducted study where conclusions cannot be drawn because of flaws in the study design or too small a sample size.

Sometimes, after looking at the data, the researcher decides that a certain comparison should be made or that it looks 'interesting'. This type of analysis is known as post hoc or data-driven, and will always carry less weight than an analysis that is pre-planned.

Box 3.12 shows the main points that should be covered in a statistical analysis plan. The analysis plan for the Early Pregnancy Study clearly states that the outcome is miscarriage before 16 weeks (box 3.13). A secondary unplanned analysis of time of miscarriage was carried out when results showed no increase in miscarriage overall, which was inconsistent with other studies that had shown an increase in the second trimester. This new analysis was reported as a secondary analysis and given less weight in the reporting of the results. Regulatory bodies such as the US Food and Drug Administration (FDA) and the UK Medicines and Healthcare products Regulatory Agency (MHRA), and many medical journals now require clinical trials to have a separate full statistical analysis plan agreed and dated before any interim or final analyses are conducted. The European Medicines Agency ICH 9 guidance provides a consensus on what this document should contain (http://www.ich.org/products/guidelines/efficacy/efficacy-single/article/statistical-principles-for-clinical-trials.html).

3.8 Required approval for research

Clinical research studies require approval from an external regulatory body such as the Institutional Review Board (IRB, United States), or the Research Ethics Committee (REC, UK). The primary aim of the regulatory process is to protect the rights and welfare of research participants, but IRBs, RECs, and their counterparts outside the US/UK also have a responsibility to ensure the scientific validity of the proposed research.

Box 3.12 Statistical analysis plan   *INFORMATION*

A statistical analysis plan should:

- State the aims of the study
- Distinguish between primary and secondary analyses
- State the outcomes to be analysed and the groups to be compared
- State methods of analysis, significance tests, and level of significance to be used
- State assumptions which need to be verified
- List confounders to be investigated and possibly adjusted for in a multifactorial model
- If there are several outcomes, describe the strategy for dealing with the possibility of spurious significant findings (type I errors)
- Describe how any missing data will be dealt with

3.8.1 The research study review process in the US and UK

In the US all research projects that involve humans must be approved by an IRB. IRBs, which consist of scientists, legal experts, and at least one person from the community, vet projects to assure ethical conduct and legal compliance. Some studies will not require a formal review by an IRB but researchers should always submit projects for approval. Further, research, especially cancer studies, may also be subject to review by an additional Scientific Review Committee (SRC). SRCs, typically comprised of local experts in a disease area, in addition to statisticians, expand the ethical requirements by demanding a rigorous review of the scientific merits of hypotheses as well as sample size and statistical power considerations.

While IRBs and SRCs rigorously protect the health and welfare of research subjects, further safeguards on patient anonymity are mandated and vigorously enforced by the US Federal Government Health Insurance Portability and Accountability Act (HIPAA). HIPAA forbids the sharing of data that can be used to identify a patient. In addition to obvious identifiers like names and medical record numbers, HIPAA also prevents the sharing of data that include dates. The US Department of Health and Human Services maintains guidelines on HIPAA and data sharing: http://www.hhs.gov/ocr/privacy/ hipaa/understanding/coveredentities/De-identification/guidance.html. Researchers should always err on the side of caution and check with local IRB officials and legal counsel before sharing any data with anyone not explicitly listed as part of the research team in an IRB-approved protocol.

In the UK, research proposals are reviewed by a committee that typically includes representation from doctors and other health professionals, biological scientists, social scientists, statisticians, and the lay public. The committee's decision can be either to approve the research, require amendments, or withhold permission for the research to take place.

In the UK the Data Protection Act 1998 covers the use of personal data and the Information Commissioner's Office is responsible for ensuring organizations meet their obligations under the Act. Healthcare organizations and research institutions are

Box 3.13 Outline statistical analysis plan   *EXAMPLE*

Early Pregnancy study

Aim

To see if bacterial vaginosis detected before 10 weeks is associated with miscarriage before 16 weeks

Study design

Cohort study

Primary outcome

Miscarriage before 16 weeks

Analysis plan

Primary analysis

The risk of miscarriage before 16 weeks with bacterial vaginosis before 10 weeks will be estimated using Cox regression, adjusting for gestational age at recruitment. Results will be presented as hazard ratios (relative risks) with 95% confidence intervals; $P < 0.05$ will be taken as significant.

Secondary analyses

The following risk factors for bacterial vaginosis will be investigated:

- Age less than 25
- Afro-Caribbean ethnic group
- Social class (3–5)
- Single marital status
- Previous oral contraception
- Smoking
- History of termination
- History of miscarriage
- History of preterm birth
- Concurrent chlamydia infection

The prevalence of bacterial vaginosis in women with and without these risk factors will be estimated and compared using hazard ratios.

Technical note

The Cox regression survival analysis approach was used in this study to allow the inclusion of all miscarriages before 16 weeks.

For further information see Oakeshott P, Kerry S, H S, Hay P. Opportunistic screening for chlamydial infection at time of cervical smear testing in general practice: prevalence study. *BMJ* 1998; 316:351–352.

Box 3.14 Choosing a funding source   *HELPFUL TIPS*

Consider the following:

+ Is the subject for this research within the priority areas for this source of funding?
+ Is the amount of funding required appropriate for the total funds available from this funding source?
+ Is the expertise of the team sufficient to carry out the work?
+ Has sufficient background work been carried out for this study (e.g. literature review, pilot studies, etc.)?

---

becoming increasingly aware of their obligations since the formation of NHS Digital (formerly HSCIC) in 2013. The NHS Digital website provides training in the use of personal data (https://www/igt.hscic.gov.uk) but you should also consult the Information Governance policies of your institution/department, and the sponsor of your study (usually the R&D office of the lead institution). Similar restrictions apply to sharing data in the UK as in the US; some institutions will have set up a Data Sharing Committee to oversee sharing of data between institutions but this is a changing and developing area.

Quantitative research will require details of the statistical aspects, such as whether a formal power calculation has been carried out, and this requires sufficient details to allow the calculations to be replicated. If the standard methods described in this chapter are used, it is not necessary to give the formulae but sufficient information must be given for someone else to check the calculations (see boxes 3.5, 3.8, and 3.10.). The example statements in this chapter (boxes 3.6, 3.7, 3.9, and 3.11) can be used as a guide. Applications for research approval that will involve statistical analyses need to provide some details about the analysis methods to be used and may be required to provide the full statistical analysis plan.

The regulatory process is more complex for intervention trials involving medicinal products than for purely observational studies. Intervention trials usually require additional registration from the appropriate national regulatory body. Guidance can be obtained from the local hospital or health institute research office.

Box 3.15 Common reasons for delay in obtaining institutional ethical approval   *HELPFUL TIPS*

+ Failure to describe the precise aims of the study and why it is important
+ Failure to demonstrate that the study will add to existing knowledge
+ Failure to justify the sample size chosen, or worse, not to specify the sample size at all
+ Poor explanation of sample size calculations so that they cannot be reproduced
+ Unclear and/or inadequate patient information sheet. This is the most common reason for delayed approval.

3.9 **When applications fail**

It is very disappointing to plan a study and then fail to get funding or institutional ethical approval. Funding is often competitive and can be subject to changes in a topic's perceived or actual priority; hence, it is difficult to give general advice on this. However, the advice given in this chapter should ensure that the statistical aspects of the study are clearly presented. Box 3.14 also gives some advice on choosing a source of funding.

If a study proposal to a funding body is rejected, there may be feedback from the review board. Reviewers may not always be right but their comments may indicate a lack of clarity in the application which can be remedied, so it is always worth taking them seriously and considering whether it is necessary to present a stronger case or to clarify some aspects. Note that the new proposal may go back to the same specialist reviewers even if the application goes to a different funding body.

Institutional ethical approval on the other hand is not competitive and studies are approved on their own merit and on the implications for patients. Box 3.15 outlines common difficulties that the authors have observed when researchers seek approval.

Box 3.16 Checklist for writing a research protocol   *CHAPTER SUMMARY*

- The aims of the research project need to be clearly written to be understood by a wide variety of people
- Sample size calculations are necessary to ensure results will be useful without putting too many people to unnecessary inconvenience or incurring unnecessary expense
- Assumptions of the calculations need to be explained and referenced where appropriate
- Writing a plan of the statistical analysis at the outset helps to ensure the aims of the study can be fulfilled and protects the validity of the results
- The role of institutional ethics committees is primarily to protect patients' welfare but they also have a responsibility for the scientific validity of the study

---

CHAPTER 4

Writing up a research study

4.1   **Introduction** *39*

4.2   **Contents of each section of the report** *39*

4.3   **Special circumstances** *46*

4.1 Introduction

A research study report may be written for any one of several different purposes, each requiring a specific format. Examples include an internal report, a report for a funding body or committee, a paper for a journal, a dissertation for an undergraduate or post-graduate degree, one of the UK Royal Medical College examinations or a thesis (e.g. PhD). The general structure is similar for all of these and follows the usual pattern for writing up the results of a scientific experiment—introduction, methods, results, and discussion (box 4.1). Exceptions are short reports and research letters, which are discussed separately in section 4.3.2. The length and relative balance of each of these sections varies according to the purpose and specified format. For example, a paper for a journal will tend to be fairly short, often less than 3000 words, whereas a dissertation may be up to 20,000 words, and a thesis considerably longer.

We outline in section 4.2 the contents of each of the sections of a research study report, with particular reference to the statistical aspects.

4.2 Contents of each section of the report

4.2.1 Abstract

The main requirement for an abstract is that it should be brief and yet be a stand-alone document. It is the first thing that most people will read and, more importantly, may be all that is read if the reader has limited time or restricted access to the full document, such as when obtaining abstracts through online journals or databases.

The abstract should state the purpose of the study and briefly describe the study design, study subjects, and the variables measured. The results section should summarize the key findings on the main variables of interest and should provide estimates of sizes of effects with confidence intervals wherever possible, as well as *P* values. Valid conclusions should be drawn without overstating or understating the interpretation of the findings. Common problems include interpreting simple associations as causal, assuming that statistical significance implies clinical significance and conversely assuming that 'not statistically

Box 4.1 Basic structure of a scientific report		*INFORMATION*
◆ Abstract	◆ Results	
◆ Background	◆ Discussion	
◆ Methods		

significant' means that there is no effect or difference. Understating conclusions is less common but some abstracts end with a statement along the lines of, 'The risk factor may be related to the disease', which probably could have been said without doing the study.

A structured abstract may be required with a specified work limit. Examples of specifications are given in box 4.2, and box 4.3 gives an example of a structured abstract.

4.2.2 Introduction

This sets the scene and describes the background to the study—what is already known about the topic, what are the gaps in knowledge, and how the proposed study will add to this. In a journal article this section is likely to be short but will be much more detailed in a dissertation, report, or thesis.

4.2.3 Methods

The purpose of the methods section is to describe the conducting of the study in sufficient detail for another researcher to be able to repeat the study. However, in a journal article as opposed to a dissertation or report, space is usually too limited for this to be possible. The use of online web-based appendices has helped to remedy this problem by allowing the brief details in a paper to be supplemented by fuller details online.

The methods section should include details of the setting or area where the study was conducted, the subjects included, the study design, technical details of any measurements made, the rationale for the chosen sample size, and the statistical methods used to analyse

Box 4.2 Examples of required structures for abstracts	*EXAMPLE*
◆ Journal: NEJM (http://www.nejm.org)	

- ◆ Journal: NEJM (http://www.nejm.org)
  - ◆ 250 words max
  - ◆ Background, Methods, Results, Conclusions
- ◆ Journal: Lancet (http://www.thelancet.com)
  - ◆ 300 words max
  - ◆ Background, Methods, Findings, Interpretation, Funding
- ◆ Conference: European Respiratory Society International Congress (https://erscongress.org/)
  - ◆ 1810 characters including spaces
  - ◆ Abstract title, Introduction or background, Aims and objectives, Methods, Results, Conclusions
  - ◆ Can include table and/or figures within allocated space

---

Box 4.3 Example of an abstract for a journal article   *EXAMPLE*

Objectives To examine changes in the emergency workload of the London Ambulance Service (LAS) between 1989 and 1999

Methods All emergency responses by the LAS during week 16 in each of 1989, 1996, and 1999 were studied. For each week, 999 call responses were analysed by time and day of call, and age/sex of the patient. Call response rates were calculated using age/sex census population estimates for London. Changes in call rates over time were calculated as rate ratios.

Results Emergency responses increased from 6624 to 13178 in the index weeks of 1989–1999. The ratio of response rates (1999/1989) was 1.91 (95% CI: 1.85, 1.96). The proportion of out-of-hours calls increased significantly from 68.8% in 1989 to 71.3% in 1999 ($P = 0.0003$). Response rates rose significantly more steeply for males than females from 1989–1999: rate ratio (95% CI); males 2.00 (1.91, 2.08), females 1.69 (1.62, 1.77), $P < 0.0001$. Response rates varied by age in each of the three years investigated. Rates were consistently highest for patients aged 75 and above, and lowest for those aged 5–14. However, there was no evidence that call rates had increased disproportionately in any particular age group ($P = 0.79$).

Conclusions Demand for emergency ambulance services in London has doubled in a decade. This increase is similar for all age groups, with no evidence of a greater rise in demand among older people. Call rates have increased more steeply in men than in women. Demographic changes do not explain the observed increases in demand.

the data. Some studies use routine data and so the description of the subjects may only need to state the time period (see box 4.3).

In other situations, subjects may be selected according to set criteria or diagnoses and these should be stated. Alternatively, the subjects may be an unselected series of available patients in a time period. However the data or subjects were selected, it is important to be able to demonstrate that the selection was done in a systematic way that will enable the study's findings to be generalized. Box 4.4 gives an example of sample description taken from the UKOS study.

The description of the study design should include the type of study; for example, cross-sectional survey, case-control, cohort, randomized controlled trial, etc. For case-control studies, the method of choosing controls and the definition of cases should be described. If cases are matched to controls then the method of matching should be described in sufficient detail to explain exactly how controls were chosen. For example, 'cases were one-to-one matched to within 2 years using the General Practice age/sex register'.

Where formal sample size calculations have been done, these should be reported (see box 4.5) and where they are inappropriate or not possible, then it is helpful to say so. Sometimes, the original sample size estimates proved to be unachievable and therefore modified estimates are made. Box 4.5 gives examples of different scenarios.

Box 4.4 Extract from a methods section describing the sample   *EXAMPLE*

Infants were eligible for the study if their gestational age was between 23 weeks and 28 weeks plus 6 days; if they were born in a participating centre; if they required endotracheal intubation from birth; and if they required ongoing intensive care. Infants were excluded if they had to be transferred to another hospital for intensive care shortly after birth or if they had a major congenital malformation.

From *The New England Journal of Medicine*, Johnson A et al., High frequency oscillatory ventilation for the prevention of chronic lung disease of prematurity, 347, 9, p. 633. Copyright © 2002 Massachusetts Medical Society. Reprinted with permission from Massachusetts Medical Society.

Chapter 3 describes how to report sample size statements in a protocol, and the same principles apply to reporting them in a paper. Further discussion of reporting sample size for a randomized clinical trial is given in chapter 12.

The report should state all statistical methods used, including methods to address missing data and any assumptions made about the data. Although the statistical package or software employed should be specified it is not enough merely to name it, as in 'the data were analysed using SPSS', or to say that 'parametric methods were used'. If the statistical method is not a standard technique, then a reference should be given. In a longer report there is room to give a full justification of the methods used; box 4.6 gives a detailed example. The report of the statistical analysis clearly states the main outcome and the predictor variables, and describes the type of data—here, categorical data in three and two categories, respectively. Then the actual analysis (chi-squared test for trend and logistic regression) is stated. Finally, the reader is told how the results will be presented (odds

---

Box 4.5 Examples of statements on sample size   *EXAMPLE*

◆ **No formal calculation but justification given**

This study was designed to be descriptive rather than analytical . . . a sample size of about 100 was feasible within the time available and was judged to be adequate to give reasonable numbers in the various categories of response expected.

◆ **Formal calculation**

The study aimed to recruit 800 babies. Assuming power of 0.9 and significance level 0.05, this was sufficient to detect a difference of 11 percentage points between treatment groups overall.

◆ **Formal calculation, later modified**

A pulmonary function subset sample size of 100 infants . . . would have enabled detection of a difference of 0.56 standard deviations between the groups, with 80% power at the 5% significance level. The achieved sample size fell below this target and, allowing for unequal group sizes, enabled detection of 0.65 standard deviations between the groups.

For further information see Bruce M, Peacock JL, Iverson A, Wolfe C. Hepatitis B and HIV antenatal screening 2: user survey. *British Journal of Midwifery* 2001; 9:640–645; Johnson AH, Peacock JL, Greenough A, Marlow N, Limb ES, Marston L et al. High-frequency oscillatory ventilation for the prevention of chronic lung disease of prematurity. *N Engl J Med* 2002; 347:633–642; and Thomas MR, Rafferty GF, Limb ES, Peacock JL, Calvert SA, Marlow N et al. Pulmonary function at follow-up of very preterm infants from the United Kingdom oscillation study. *Am J Respir Crit Care Med* 2004; 169:868–872.

Table 4.1 Baseline characteristics of a sample   *EXAMPLE*

Characteristics of study group: 230 pregnant women who missed antenatal clinic appointments

Variable	No.	Mean (SD) or %
Age (years)	229	26.1 (5.5)
Height (cm)	225	161.6 (6.3)
Weight (kg)	225	61.7 (10.4)
Alcohol (g/week)	230	17.3 (33.6)
Birthweight of baby (g)	229	3280 (477)
Marital status		
Married	156	69%
Single	59	26%
Widowed/separated/divorced	12	5%
Total	227	100%
Social class		
Non-manual	90	43%
Manual	117	57%
Total	207	100%
Education		
Minimum	137	61%
More than minimum	88	39%
Total	225	100%
Current smoking		
Smoker	118	52%
Non-smoker	110	48%
Total	228	100%

ratios and 95% confidence intervals) and what statistical package was used. Further examples of how to describe specific statistical methods are given throughout the book.

Sometimes the researcher may not know in advance exactly which methods will be used, as this can depend on early findings. In such circumstances it is not obvious whether to include these in the 'methods' section as if they were determined in advance, or to describe them in the 'results' section. We advise that all methods are described in the methods section if at all possible, unless the text flows better if they are included with the results.

4.2.4 Results

The results section should begin by describing the basic characteristics of the study population. This should include the total numbers of subjects or observations with a breakdown of these numbers to show the reasons for missing data, e.g. refusal, non-response, dropout, data not recorded, etc. If the study is comparing groups, as in a randomized trial, then baseline data for the groups should be given. If there is a lot of information it may be

---

Box 4.6 Describing the statistical methods _EXAMPLE_

Description of study

This example comes from a study which aimed to investigate the association between self-reported domestic violence and health in primary school children. The survey consisted of a self-completion questionnaire.

The main predictor was self-reported exposure to domestic violence in three categories. The outcome variables were aspects of health care use, health behaviour, and social support.

Description of statistical analysis

The outcome was self-reported physical violence at home in the last month, with three categories of exposure: 'none', 'once or twice', and 'often'. The health outcomes included questions on healthcare use, health-related behaviours, and social support and were analysed as binary variables.

The chi-squared test for trend was used to analyse the differences in proportions of health-related outcomes in the three violence exposure categories. Multivariable logistic regression was used to investigate the association between violence and health outcomes, after adjustment for socio-economic status. Results are presented as unadjusted and adjusted odds ratios with 95% confidence intervals. Data were analysed using Stata and in-house software.

For further information see Stewart G, Ruggles R, Peacock J. The association of self-reported violence at home and health in primary school pupils in West London. _J Public Health_ 2004; 26:19–23.

---

easier for the reader to assimilate if these data are presented in a table, but where there are many baseline variables the choice of which to present is a matter of judgement. Table 4.1 gives an example of summarizing a subset of data from a larger sample. The authors have previously used this as a teaching exercise to illustrate how different types of data can be incorporated into just one table. (We noticed that less experienced students and researchers tended to put each variable in a separate table, which not only wasted space but also made the results rather disjointed.) Guidelines on how to describe baseline characteristics can be found in chapter 5.

The main results of statistical analyses can often be summarized in tables and graphs. Missing data should be accounted for wherever possible so that the numbers 'add up'. Often totals will vary from table to table by a small amount, either because data are missing for that variable or because subjects do not answer a particular question. In such cases it is usually sufficient to give the maximum total and then to say, 'numbers vary slightly from table to table due to missing data'.

It is often easier to assimilate several sets of numbers when they are in table form rather than given in the text. This is certainly possible when writing a report, dissertation, or thesis, where there is usually space to include many tables. However, this may not be possible when writing a journal article, as there may be a limit to the number of tables allowed. The text itself should describe and summarize the important features in terms of the sizes of effects, the differences between groups, or the strengths of associations, etc., as appropriate.

Box 4.7 Possible statistical issues for inclusion in the discussion   *HELPFUL TIPS*

- Size of effects observed, width of CIs
- Consequences of multiple testing
- Limitations of methods of analysis
- Limitations due to design e.g. interpretation of non-randomized intervention studies
- Known and unknown confounding
- Effects of missing data
- Accuracy of measurements made—random error/bias
- Future work, new data, further analyses

It is unnecessary to repeat information, such as a difference, its confidence interval, and *P* value, when that information is already presented in tables.

4.2.5 Discussion

Many aspects of the discussion will centre on interpreting the findings in the context of previous work and current knowledge. Such discussion may not be intrinsically statistical. However, there are several statistical issues which may require discussion or comment. Box 4.7 lists some of these.

It can be useful to set the sizes of effects and widths of confidence intervals in the context of current knowledge. Box 4.8 gives an example from a study of the adverse health effects of outdoor air pollution, which had, in general, found very similar effect sizes to those previously reported by others. For this particular outcome the estimate was higher than one reported previously, but the current study's 95% confidence interval was wide. Hence, the two studies' findings were not inconsistent with each other.

In some studies, many hypothesis tests are performed, increasing the possibility of spurious significant results (type 1 errors). Where a single and unexpected significant result has been found it is sensible to view this cautiously and discuss the possibility that it is a false positive finding. This problem is common in exploratory studies.

Sometimes there are unavoidable limitations in the design or statistical analysis used. This can often happen with student projects where there are tight time constraints, but may

---

Box 4.8 Example of the statistical interpretation of results in the discussion section   *EXAMPLE*

Our findings were of greater magnitude than those observed by Hoek and others . . . (who) reported a 3% increase . . . our estimate was equivalent to a 13% increase in risk, but the 95% confidence interval was wide: −8% to +36%.

For further information see Peacock JL, Symonds P, Jackson P, Bremner SA, Scarlett JF, Strachan DP et al. Acute effects of winter air pollution on respiratory function in schoolchildren in southern England. *Occup Environ Med* 2003; 60:82–89.

also happen with other studies. In such cases any limitations and their potential implications should be clearly described and discussed. In practice, no study is perfect and all have some limitations. In a well-designed study, the limitations will be outweighed by the strengths, and the results will be robust.

4.3 Special circumstances

4.3.1 Writing abstracts for conferences

Like abstracts for reports, abstracts for oral and poster conference presentations must stand alone, because conference abstracts in particular are often published in their own right. The specification for these abstracts varies from conference to conference but may be structured and will almost certainly have a word or character limit (box 4.2).

4.3.2 Short reports and research letters

Some journals allow authors to submit short reports or research letters, which are typically 500–1000 words in length with only one table or figure allowed. They do not always fit the usual structure and sections, such as introduction and methods, can be combined. It can be difficult to write for this type of format because of these constraints but it is ideal for a small piece of work.

Box 4.9 Check list for writing up a research study　　*CHAPTER SUMMARY*

Abstract
- Stand-alone document
- Report main outcome with estimates and 95% CI if possible
- Draw valid conclusions

Introduction
- What is the research question?
- What do we know already?
- What are the gaps?
- What does this study add?

Methods
- Describe study design and conduct
- Choice of subjects
- Sample size
- Data collected
- Statistical analysis

Results
- Describe characteristics of the sample
- Describe findings
- Don't just give P values—present estimates and CIs

Box 4.9 *continued*

Discussion

- Summarize findings
- Describe how they fit with existing knowledge
- Discuss any limitations
- Draw conclusions and make suggestions for future research

CHAPTER 5

Introduction to presenting statistical analyses

5.1   **Introduction** *48*
5.2   **Presenting numerical data** *48*
5.3   **Beginning the results section** *49*
5.4   **Describing the results of the recruitment process** *49*
5.5   **Assessing non-response bias** *51*
5.6   **Presenting the results for different media** *52*
5.7   **Drawing up a profile of a group of subjects** *56*
5.8   **Drawing graphs** *56*
5.9   **Using text to refer to tables and graphs** *57*
5.10 **Presenting categorical data** *58*
5.11 **Presenting continuous data** *58*

5.1 Introduction

This chapter shows how to present descriptive statistical analyses, including how to display the results of the recruitment process and how to describe the characteristics of the study sample. Guidelines are laid out for the presentation of numerical data, such as percentages, *P* values, confidence intervals, etc., and for presenting tables and graphs, with examples given to draw out the general principles. We show how to present different types of data, such as continuous and binary data, and also make recommendations for presentation for different media, such as papers, dissertations and theses, and oral presentations.

5.2 Presenting numerical data

It is important to present numerical data clearly, accurately, and concisely, so that the message that the data contain is communicated. This is not always straightforward, especially when extracting results from computer packages where many details may be provided and where results are given to a high level of precision. For example, statistical packages will usually present a mean to many decimal places. However, if the original data are recorded as whole numbers, then it is misleading to present a mean to several decimal places, as it suggests a spuriously high level of accuracy—one decimal place is sufficient. Similarly, percentages should not be given to more than one decimal place if the actual frequencies are also stated. Apart from false precision, the other reason for giving fewer decimal places is to help the reader assimilate the information. A table of means or percentages which is presented with several decimal places is hard to absorb.

The other reason for being selective in presentation is that statistical packages often produce detailed output of the statistical procedures used, and not all of the details need reporting. Further, in particular contexts not all of the results may make sense and so the reader has to select carefully which to present. We give many examples in this book, advising which data to select and present from SAS, Stata, R, and SPSS outputs. For example, where arithmetic, geometric, and harmonic means are given by a statistical package, it is likely that only one will be needed and reported (see section 5.11.2).

The presentation of P values can cause some difficulty. The actual P value should usually be given, whether or not the results are statistically significant. Two significant figures are sufficient. Sometimes packages give very small P values as '$P = 0.0000$'. This does not mean that the P value equals zero but that the calculated P value is smaller than 0.0001 and is therefore 0.0000, to four decimal places. We recommend presenting this as $P < 0.0001$ rather than $P = 0.0000$. Similarly, '$P = 1.0000$' does not mean that the P value is exactly 1, but that it is 1.0000, to four decimal places and we recommend presenting this as $P > 0.999$. Box 5.1 gives a summary of guidelines for a range of statistics.

5.3 Beginning the results section

Before performing the main analyses it is important to describe how the sample was obtained and the main relevant characteristics of that sample. The actual recruitment methodology should be described in the methods section of a paper (see section 4.2.3) but the numbers of patients actually recruited, response rates, and reasons for non-response should be described at the beginning of the results section. As well as giving the numbers of subjects, it is often useful to describe key characteristics of the group which might affect the interpretation of the results or the extent to which the results may be generalized to other patient groups.

5.4 Describing the results of the recruitment process

Box 5.2 gives the key points to consider when describing the results of the recruitment process, from the sampling frame through to the patients included in the analysis. This allows the reader to assess whether the results are likely to be biased in any way and also demonstrates that the study has been carefully carried out and that the results can be trusted.

For all randomized trials a flowchart should be included as recommended in the CONSORT guidelines (see chapter 12). However, a flow chart can be useful for other studies too. In the Wandsworth Heart and Stroke Study, 3606 patients were initially selected from nine General Practice lists but only 1577 patients were included in the analysis. Figure 5.1 shows a flowchart illustrating the steps taking place between when the sample is chosen and the final data analysed. Many patients had moved away and so would not have

---

Box 5.1 Presenting numerical data and common statistics　　　*HELPFUL TIPS*

Proportions
- Give to two significant figures (e.g. 0.25, 0.0056)
- Give numbers as well as the actual proportion unless obvious
- Use percentage or rate per 1000, 10,000, etc., if proportion is very small

Percentages
- Give percentages less than 10, or greater than 90, to one decimal place (e.g. 5.2%, 93.8%)
- Consider giving percentages between 10% and 90% as whole numbers, unless the extra precision is needed (e.g. 27% vs 27.3%)
- Give numbers as well as actual percentage unless obvious but make clear which is which
- Do not use percentages if sample is less than 10

Mean, SD, SE
- Present to one more significant figure than original data
- Do not use +/− or ± as this is potentially ambiguous
  Use 'mean (SD) = . . .' or 'mean (SE) = . . .'

CIs
- Present to one more significant figure than original data
- Present as 'x to y' or 'x, y', not 'x–y', since ambiguous if negative values are possible

P values
- Present actual P values wherever possible, whether significant or not
- Give no more than two significant figures, e.g.0.0392 → 0.039, 0.596 → 0.60
- If package gives 'P = 0.0000', present as P < 0.0001
- If package gives 'P = 1.0000', present as P > 0.999

* or ** or ***
- Not necessary if the actual P value is given
- Can be useful where space is limited and CIs are given
- Indicate statistical significance at different levels
- Usual meaning: *P < 0.05, **P < 0.01, ***P < 0.001

Notes
- *Significant figures* are non-zero digits; e.g. 0.00568 to two significant figures is 0.0057
- *Decimal places* are the number of digits after the decimal point; e.g. 0.00568 to two decimal places is 0.01. Retain right-hand 0s, e.g. 3.02 to one decimal place is 3.0, not 3
- *Select* appropriate results from computer output and edit for presentation. Results provided in computer output may not all be relevant in a given context
- *Retain* more significant figures than suggested above when figures will be used for further calculations to maintain accuracy (retain all if in doubt)
- *Rules for rounding 5s:* 0.0325 → 0.033, 0.0324 → 0.032

**Box 5.2 Key points in describing the results of the
                  recruitment process**   *INFORMATION*

- Sampling frame
- Number of subjects originally selected
- Number of subjects subsequently excluded because of ineligibility
- Number of non-responders
- Reasons for non-response, if known
- Comparison of responders and non-responders, if possible
- Number of subjects withdrawing before completing the study

been included had the lists been up to date, and hence were removed before the response rate was calculated. Giving all the numbers provides a clear audit trail and shows that the response rate is probably an underestimate, as some of those who did not reply may also have moved away.

5.5 **Assessing non-response bias**

We have to accept that every person has the right to refuse to take part in medical research but the resulting effects on the results should not be ignored. As much information on

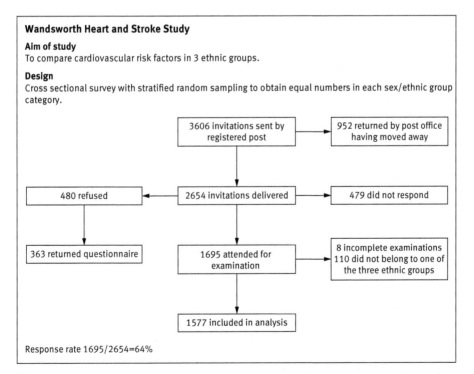

Wandsworth Heart and Stroke Study

Aim of study
To compare cardiovascular risk factors in 3 ethnic groups.

Design
Cross sectional survey with stratified random sampling to obtain equal numbers in each sex/ethnic group category.

3606 invitations sent by registered post → 952 returned by post office having moved away

2654 invitations delivered

480 refused ← 2654 invitations delivered → 479 did not respond

363 returned questionnaire

1695 attended for examination → 8 incomplete examinations / 110 did not belong to one of the three ethnic groups

1577 included in analysis

Response rate 1695/2654=64%

🔲 **Figure 5.1** Flowchart of the recruitment process for the Wandsworth Heart and Stroke Study

---

Box 5.3 Assessing non-response bias   *EXAMPLE*

Wandsworth Heart and Stroke Study

Table **Number of patients recruited by sex and ethnic groups (N = 1577)**

	Males	Females
White	233	290
African origin	208	341
Asian	253	252

- 500 patients in each sex and ethnic group were selected from the sampling frame
- The table shows that, of those that took part, there was an excess of women of African origin

For further information see Cappuccio FP, Cook DG, Atkinson RW, Strazzullo P. Prevalence, detection, and management of cardiovascular risk factors in different ethnic groups in south London. *Heart* 1997; 78:555–563.

---

non-responders as possible should be obtained to allow potential bias due to non-response to be assessed. Box 5.3 shows that in the Wandsworth Heart and Stroke Study more women than men agreed to take part, possibly because of the difficulty in attending for the research interview during the working day. In addition, some subjects who refused to attend for examination agreed to complete a postal questionnaire. The replies to this questionnaire can be used to further assess non-response bias.

5.6 Presenting the results for different media

The way in which the results are presented will depend on whether you are giving a talk, preparing a poster, writing a paper for a scientific journal, or writing a dissertation or thesis.

Reports, dissertations, and theses are usually fairly long and require the results to be presented in detail. Box 5.4 shows an extract from a report of a study into the role of x-rays in the management of lower back pain in primary care, and describes the characteristics of the patients recruited.

Papers for journals usually have word limits, but need to contain sufficient information for the reader to critically appraise the study. Therefore, results need to be presented very concisely, usually in tables and text, rather than in graphs. Table 5.1 shows how a single table can display a lot of information very concisely. The prevalences of bacterial vaginosis in women with and without each characteristic are shown side by side, so they can be compared. The most appropriate comparison statistics is the ratio of the prevalences (the relative risk), and this is shown alongside the relative risk, adjusting for age. (This analysis was carried out using the Cox proportional hazards model—see chapter 11.) By setting the unadjusted and adjusted relative risks side by side, the effect of adjustment can be easily seen. In this way, a considerable amount of information can be summarized in one table.

Graphs in papers should only be used when really necessary to convey information that cannot be presented satisfactorily in tables—usually when we want to plot the actual data values, such as in a scattergram (e.g. figure 9.1), or to plot individual study results in a meta-analysis (chapter 13).

Box 5.4 Population profile from a report *EXAMPLE*

Low Back Pain Study

Aim of study To assess the effect of early x-rays for low back pain.

Design Observational study and a randomized controlled trial.

Patients characteristics The average age of the patients was 41.8 years, and 52% were women. Pain had been present for less than one week in 28% of patients and more than 6 months in 22% (table 1). The mean number of consultations in the year before recruitment was 4.0, compared to a national average of 3.8. The level of pain experienced by these patients is shown in table 2.

Table 1 **Length of present episode of back pain**

	Number of % patients	(n=548)
Less than 1 week	156	28
1–4 weeks	156	28
4 weeks to <8 weeks	55	10
8 weeks to <6 months	59	11
6 months and over	122	22

Table 2 **Level of pain experienced at recruitment**

	Number of % patients	(n=555)
No pain at all	6	1
Little pain	67	12
Moderate pain	205	37
Quite bad pain	155	28
Very bad pain	101	18
Almost unbearable pain	21	4

For further information see Kerry S, Oakeshott P, Dundas D, Williams J. Influence of postal distribution of the Royal College of Radiologists' guidelines, together with feedback on radiological referral rates, on X-ray referrals from general practice: a randomized controlled trial. *Fam Pract* 2000; 17:46–52.

The purpose of oral presentations and posters is to convey a key message quickly. Simple tables and graphs are usually more appropriate than complicated tables and solid text. It will often be necessary to omit some of the details from tables that would be presented in a paper. Table 5.2 shows a simplified version of the table in table 5.1 that would be suitable for a poster or slide. Alternatively the results could be displayed graphically, as in figure 5.2. The level of pain experienced by patients recruited to the Low Back Pain Study that was presented in a table in box 5.4 is shown as a graph in figure 5.3.

Table 5.1 Single concise table from a paper with unadjusted and adjusted estimates   *EXAMPLE*

Early Pregnancy Study

Characteristics of 1201 newly pregnant women according to bacterial vaginosis status at recruitment

Characteristic	No. (%) with characteristic	Prevalence (proportion) of women with bacterial vaginosis among women:		Relative risk (95% CI)	Relative risk (95% CI) adjusted for age
		With characteristic	Without characteristic		
Age <25 (n=1201)	150 (13)	23 (34/150)	13 (140/1051)	1.7 (1.2, 2.5) **	-
Black Caribbean or Black African (n=1096)	116 (11)	34 (39/116)	11 (109/980)	3.0 (2.1, 4.4) ***	2.9 (2.0, 4.2) ***
Social class 3 to 5[1] (n=1036)	415 (40)	16 (68/415)	10 (65/621)	1.6 (1.1, 2.2) **	1.5 (1.0, 2.1) *
Single, widowed, or divorced (n=1095)	94 (9)	29 (27/94)	12 (116/1001)	2.5 (1.6, 3.8) ***	2.3 (1.5, 3.7) ***
Previous contraception oral or none (n=1084)	682 (63)	15 (101/682)	11 (43/402)	1.4 (0.97, 2.0)	1.4 (0.97, 2.0)
No previous pregnancies (n=1094)	388 (35)	11 (43/388)	15 (107/706)	0.73 (0.51, 1.0)	0.73 (0.51, 1.0)
Previous termination of pregnancy (n=1087)	270 (25)	22 (59/270)	11 (87/817)	2.1 (1.5, 2.9) ***	2.0 (1.5, 2.8) ***

[1]For women who were unemployed or students, partner's social class was used when available.
*P < 0.05, **P < 0.01, ***P < 0.001.

Description

Results section

Bacterial vaginosis was more common in younger women, those of African origin, in lower social classes, and those with a history of termination of pregnancy.

For further information see Oakeshott P, Hay P, Hay S, Steinke F, Rink E, Thomas B et al. Detection of Chlamydia trachomatis infection in early pregnancy using self-administered vaginal swabs and first pass urines: a cross-sectional community-based survey. *Br J Gen Pract* 2002; 52:830–832.

Table 5.2 Table suitable for an oral presentation   *EXAMPLE*

Table **Relative risk of bacterial vaginosis in 1201 pregnant women**

Risk factor	Relative risk of bacterial vaginosis
Age <25	1.7 (1.2, 2.5)**
Afro-Caribbean or Black African	3.0 (2.1, 4.4)***
Social class 3 to 5	1.6 (1.1, 2.2)**
Single, widowed, or divorced	2.5 (1.6, 3.8)***
No previous pregnancies	0.7 (0.5, 1.0)
Previous termination of pregnancy	2.1 (1.5, 2.9)***

***P < 0.001, **P < 0.01.

Care should be taken, when preparing slides for oral presentations, not to make the font size too small and so difficult to read. This in itself will, of course, restrict the amount of information that can be presented. In addition, it may be less distracting for the audience to be presented with small amounts of information at one time, and so several simple slides may be better than one complicated one.

Posters need to be attractive and eye-catching—if the poster does not quickly gain the interest of the viewer, there is a danger that they will simply walk past. Graphs are a useful way of presenting key findings in a colourful way so that the main message can be understood easily.

Boxes 5.5 and 5.6 give a list of guidelines to consider when deciding how to present data in graphs and tables. These will help to ensure the graph or table is clear to the audience. We recommend using two-dimensional rather than three-dimensional graphs, as it is difficult to read numbers and percentages on the scale when 3-D is used.

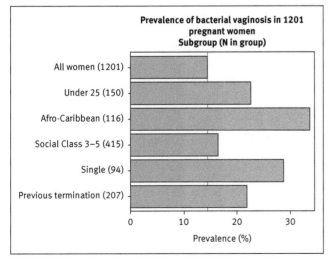

Figure 5.2 Several binary variables on one graph suitable for a poster or talk (SAS)

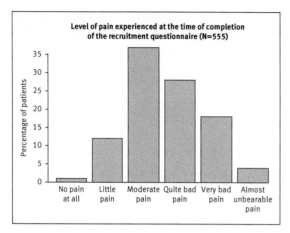

Figure 5.3 Graph for a ordered categorical variable suitable for poster or talk (R)

5.7 Drawing up a profile of a group of subjects

Many studies are comparative and hence the presentation of results will focus on the comparison between the groups. However, it is useful to start with a simple description of some of the main features of the sample, e.g. how old they were and the percentage of females, as well as some key variables relevant to the subject of interest. Box 5.4 gives an example taken from a report of a study.

A more concise profile of a group of subjects, written for inclusion in a paper, is shown in box 5.7. It gives the ages of the women and other pertinent factors, setting the scene before the paper continues with a description of the risk factors for bacterial vaginosis (table 5.1).

5.8 Drawing graphs

Graphs can be drawn in SAS, R, Stata, or SPSS and imported into word-processing or presentation documents, (e.g. Word or PowerPoint). Some people use Excel for graphs, as it is

---

Box 5.5 Guidelines for graphs   *HELPFUL TIPS*

- Title should explain what the graph is about and which subjects or observations are included
- Give number of subjects or observations
- Label axes, giving units as appropriate
- Refer to graph in the text
- Does the graph show enough information to justify the space it takes?
- For clarity, use two-dimensional rather than three-dimensional graphs
- For a paper: is a graph necessary? Could the data be presented in another way?
- In a slide or poster: will the text be legible?

Box 5.6 Guidelines for tables   *HELPFUL TIPS*

- Title should explain what table is about and which subjects or observations are included
- Give number of subjects or observations overall and by group where appropriate
- Label rows and columns clearly
- Give confidence intervals for comparisons, not just P values
- Give SD, SE, or CI for means
- Give percentages alongside frequencies unless group size is less than 10
- Give range or interquartile range for medians
- State units used
- Use consistent and appropriate decimal places
- Refer to table in the text
- Keep table simple for a slide or poster and check text size for legibility

---

commonly available, inputting the summary values from a statistics package. Alternatively, there are specialist graphics packages available.

5.9 Using text to refer to tables and graphs

All tables and graphs should be referred to in the text. It is also advisable to indicate the key findings of the table, as illustrated in box 5.4. This is more helpful to the reader than 'the results are presented in the table(s)'. The text indicates the message; the data in the table support the statement in the text. The same information should not be presented in both tables and graphs, and the text should support rather than repeat the tables and graphs.

Box 5.7 Profile of a group of subjects from a short report in a journal   *EXAMPLE*

Early Pregnancy study

Between June 1998 and July 2000, 1216 pregnant women, mean age 31 (range 16–48), were recruited; 1126 were from general practices, and 90 from family planning clinics. The median gestation at recruitment was 49 days (range 12–69). Ascertainment of pregnancy outcome at 16 weeks was 99.8% (1214 of 1216). Of the 1107 women who responded to the questionnaire, 78% (867) described their ethnicity as white, 7% (75) as Afro-Caribbean, 4% (44) as Black African, 6% (65) as of Indian subcontinent origin, and 5% (56) as other ethnic groups.

For further information see Oakeshott P, Hay P, Hay S, Steinke F, Rink E, Thomas B et al. Detection of Chlamydia trachomatis infection in early pregnancy using self-administered vaginal swabs and first pass urines: a cross-sectional community-based survey. *Br J Gen Pract* 2002; 52:830–832.

5.10 Presenting categorical data

5.10.1 Tables for categorical data

Box 5.4 gives an example of a table for an ordered categorical variable, the amount of pain that was experienced. Numbers of subjects in each category are given with the percentages. It is useful to give percentages unless the total number in the sample is very small, say, less than 10, when numbers alone will suffice. Providing percentages in this case gives the impression of spurious accuracy. Several variables can be presented in the same table, one underneath the other. This concisely conveys information together in one table.

Often researchers re-group ordered categories into two. This has its drawbacks, particularly if the categories are decided upon after looking at the data, and it does discard information. However, it can be useful if conciseness is important. In the UK Royal College of Radiologists' guidelines concerning x-rays for lower back pain, x-rays were not recommended for patients who had been in pain for less than 8 weeks except under certain circumstances. The 'length of episode' variable was therefore grouped into 'less than 8 weeks' and '8 weeks or more' for further analysis.

Where there are only two categories, i.e. binary variables, it is unnecessary to give the numbers in both categories; instead only one category need be presented. This makes tables and graphs more concise and easier to absorb. For example, figure 5.2 simply shows the percentages with bacterial vaginosis, and does not show the percentages without.

5.10.2 Graphs for categorical data

Ordered categories can be presented in a bar chart (figure 5.3). Where we wish to compare two groups of subjects these can be presented as bar in a different colour or shading alongside (figure 5.4). Several binary variables can be presented on one bar chart (figure 5.2). The graphs shown here have enough information for one slide of a presentation without containing so much information that it is difficult to absorb quickly.

5.11 Presenting continuous data

5.11.1 Tables and text

Continuous variables are usually summarized by an average, either the mean or the median. A measure of spread of the observations (standard deviation, range, or interquartile range)

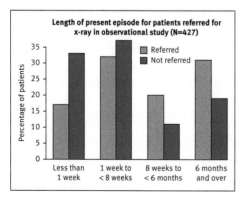

Figure 5.4 Graph containing two groups of patients suitable for poster or talk (R)

or a measure of accuracy (standard error or confidence interval) should be given along-side. Box 5.8 gives some tips on which of these to choose. When quoting standard errors or standard deviations it is important to specify which has been used. The commonly used notation +/− is best avoided and replaced by mean (SD) or mean (SE). For example, 'mean (SD) systolic blood pressure was 121 (19)'. Petrie and Sabin 2009 gives a useful list of advantages and disadvantages of the various measures.

When presenting confidence intervals it is preferable to use the word 'to' for separating the two values rather than a 'dash'. A dash is confusing where negative values are possible since the dash looks the same as a minus sign. Separating the values by a comma is favoured by some journals and is useful if space is limited.

The choice of statistics (e.g. mean or median) should reflect the type of analysis to be carried out. For example, when using a *t* test which compares two means, it is useful to present the means being compared. Analysis of variance and multiple regression are extensions of the *t* test, and therefore it would be consistent to present means for these analyses. A median is the middle rank and hence is more appropriate when rank tests are being used, such as a Mann—Whitney *U* test.

5.11.2 Presenting transformed data

Sometimes the data are highly skewed but taking the logarithm (often abbreviated to 'log') of the values produces a distribution which is near Normal. In this case we may wish to do the statistical analysis on the log transformed data (see sections 7.3.2 and 8.2.2 for

---

Box 5.8 When to present standard deviation, standard error, or a confidence interval *HELPFUL TIPS*

Standard deviation

- Good descriptor of the distribution of the data values
- Use where the variability of the data values is of interest
- Use when estimating reference ranges
- Can be useful for assessing whether assumptions of the *t* test hold (see section 7.3)
- Can be difficult to interpret for skewed data

Standard error

- Measures precision of an estimate
- Related to the confidence interval
- Precision is more clearly indicated by the confidence interval, but can report standard error if space limited
- Cannot be used where data are transformed then back-transformed

Confidence interval

- Shows the precision of an estimate, e.g. mean, proportion, relative risk, etc.
- Generally preferable for reporting to standard error (see the previous category)
- Can be calculated for log-transformed data (geometric mean—back-transformed mean of log transformed data)

examples). However, the log data will be difficult for readers to interpret, and should be back-transformed by anti-logging (i.e. taking the exponential), to get back to the original scale. Log transforming data, calculating a mean, and then back-transforming gives the geometric mean. This is equivalent to taking the nth root of the product of all the n original observations. Sometimes back-transformation needs to be done by hand on a calculator, while at other times the statistical analysis package may produce the back-transformed results. In Stata, geometric means and their confidence intervals can be calculated directly as in figure 5.5, while in SPSS the results need to be back-transformed on a calculator.

Note that data with skewed distribution, which follows a Normal distribution after log transformation, is sometimes referred to as following a 'log Normal distribution'.

Other transformations can also be used such as the square root and reciprocal and angular transforms. Like the log transform, these transformations also lead to problems in interpreting effect sizes. The choice of transformation depends on the degree of skewedness, and the requirement to have an estimate of effect and confidence interval. Further discussion is beyond the scope of this book but more details are given in Bland 2015 (chapter 10).

5.11.3 Presenting different types of data in one table

It can be useful to be able to present all variables with a common theme in one table. Table 5.3 shows the cardiovascular risk variables measured in the Wandsworth Heart and Stroke Study and includes continuous variables, untransformed and transformed, and categorical

---

The variable *hdl* is HDL cholesterol and is positively skewed. It therefore was 'log transformed' to give Normally distributed data. Analysis is on the log transformation of *hdl*, named loghdl. After analysis the results are usually back-transformed to the original units by taking the exponential. In Stata the **means** command calculates the geometric mean equivalent to the exponential of the mean of the transformed data. The following example shows these are the same. Note that the 'log' is to base e.

```
. use "c"\Projects\Books\Presenting\data\statadata\hdl.dta", clear

. gen loghdl = log (hdl)
(108 missing values generated)

. ci loghdl
```

Variable	Obs	Mean	Std. Err.	[95% Conf. Interval]	
loghdl	1469	.2734075	.0076731	.258356	.288459

```
. means hdl
```

Variable	Type	Obs	Mean	[95% Conf. Interval]	
hdl	Arithmetic	1469	1.372298	1.35127	1.393326
	Geometric	1469	1.314436	1.2948	1.33437
	Harmonic	1469	1.258455	1.239012	1.278518

log(1.2948) = 0.258356

Figure 5.5 Calculating the confidence interval of a geometric mean (Stata)

Table 5.3 Presenting several types of variables with a common theme in one table   *EXAMPLE*

Table **Age-adjusted means (95% confidence interval) for cardiovascular risk factors in men from the Wandsworth Heart and Stroke Study (n = 694)**

Variable	Mean (95% CI)
Age (years)	50.6 (50.2 to 51.0)
Systolic blood pressure (mm Hg)	131 (129 to 132)
Diastolic blood pressure (mm Hg)	83 (82 to 84)
Total cholesterol (mmol/l)	5.8 (5.7 to 5.9)
HDL cholesterol (mmol/l)[1]	1.18 (1.15 to 1.20)
Current smoking (%)	28 (25 to 31)
Diabetes (%)	14 (11 to 16)

[1] Geometric mean.

Notes
- All results are presented with 95% confidence intervals
- Smoking and diabetes are binary, and expressed as percentages, indicated with a '%' sign
- HDL cholesterol is skewed and so log transformed for analysis. The back-transformed mean is the geometric mean

variables. Smoking and diabetes have been included as the percentage of patients smoking and the percentage with diabetes, respectively. Arithmetic means have been used for blood pressure, but HDL cholesterol was log transformed for analysis, and so the geometric mean has been presented, with this indicated in a footnote. Another example of presenting several types of data with a common theme is given in table 4.1.

5.11.4 Presenting continuous data in graphs

Often we use graphs such as histograms and Normal plots to assess the nature of a distribution, i.e. whether it is skewed or symmetric, and for identifying any outliers (e.g. figure 2.4). These are useful tools for verifying assumptions about the data, as in sections 7.2 and 8.2, but are not usually presented in a paper due to lack of space. In a dissertation or thesis the graphs might be useful to help explain the methodology; for example, to justify why the data were transformed.

Graphs may be useful if the distribution of a key continuous variable is of interest; for example, when calculating a Normal range, or when comparing the distribution of the data with a predefined cut-off. Figure 5.6 shows the distribution of systolic blood pressure among all subjects in the Wandsworth Heart and Stroke Study, with the cut-off of 140 mm Hg indicated by shading the graph. This cut-off is commonly used to define hypertension.

Another situation where the distribution itself rather than the mean is of key interest is in the age/sex profile of a country. This can be shown as a population pyramid, which is similar to a histogram but using the vertical axis for age (figure 5.7). In the communities studied in rural Ghana a large proportion of the population was under 20 and there were fewer men in their

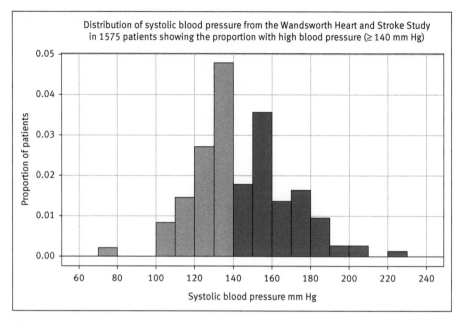

Figure 5.6 Using a graph to compare a distribution with a cut-off (R)

20s and 30s than women. This is a rural population and the men may have migrated to work. Population pyramids from African nations now show a lack of men and women in their 20s, 30s, and 40s due to the AIDS epidemic. Such trends cannot be deduced from the mean and standard deviations alone.

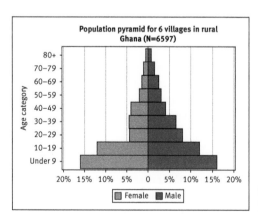

Figure 5.7 Displaying two histograms: A population pyramid

Box 5.9 Presenting statistical analyses   *CHAPTER SUMMARY*

- Be careful and selective in presenting numerical data especially when extracting results from computer output
- Tables and graphs need to be clear so they stand alone
- Graphs need to convey sufficient information to justify the space they require
- Present results concisely in papers, concentrating on tables and text, and only using graphs where information cannot be presented in a table
- Use simple tables and graphs for oral presentations and posters.
- Before doing the main statistical analysis:
    - Describe the results of the recruitment process from the selection of subjects through to the analysis
    - Draw up a profile of the subjects recruited

CHAPTER 6

Single group studies

6.1   **Introduction** *64*

6.2   **Prevalence studies** *64*

6.3   **Presenting the results of prevalence studies** *65*

6.4   **Screening and diagnostic studies: Sensitivity and specificity** *66*

6.5   **Presentation of sensitivity and specificity** *67*

6.6   **Comment on results** *67*

6.7   **Screening studies for rare conditions** *68*

6.8   **Extensions to sensitivity and specificity** *70*

6.9   **Further reading** *70*

6.1 Introduction

Single group studies are often descriptive rather than analytical and aim to produce estimates of quantities, such as the prevalence of a condition or the sensitivity and specificity of a screening test, or a reference range for a measurement. In such studies it is particularly important to describe how the sample was chosen, the characteristics of the sample, and how the outcomes were defined and measured.

For example, the prevalence of hypertension may vary according to how many blood pressure measurements are taken, with a lower prevalence being obtained when three measurements are taken compared with two, since an individual's lowest value is taken as the 'true' reading. However, if we wish to investigate whether blood pressure is related to body mass index, a systematic bias in the measurement of blood pressure is unlikely to affect the relationship between the two variables. Finally, we note that a measure of precision, such as a confidence interval, should be given as well as the proportions themselves.

This chapter describes how to present prevalence studies and the results of screening studies.

6.2 Prevalence studies

To illustrate data presentation in prevalence studies we use the chlamydia study that was previously shown in chapter 3. The study's aim was to estimate the prevalence of chlamydial infection in women aged 16–34 who were having cervical smear tests in Inner London General Practices.

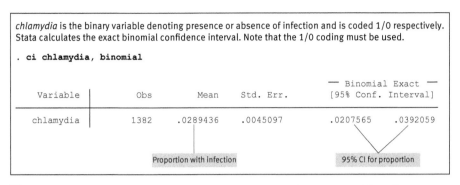

chlamydia is the binary variable denoting presence or absence of infection and is coded 1/0 respectively. Stata calculates the exact binomial confidence interval. Note that the 1/0 coding must be used.

```
. ci chlamydia, binomial
```

				— Binomial Exact —
Variable	Obs	Mean	Std. Err.	[95% Conf. Interval]
chlamydia	1382	.0289436	.0045097	.0207565 .0392059

Proportion with infection

95% CI for proportion

Figure 6.1 Output for calculating a prevalence and 95% confidence interval (Stata)

Figure 6.1 shows the Stata output, which calculates the proportion of women with the infection, and a 95% confidence interval.

There is no straightforward way to calculate a 95% confidence interval for a single proportion in SPSS, so users can either do the calculation using a calculator and the relevant formula (see Peacock and Peacock 2011 (page 244)) or can use another statistical programme such as CIPROPORTION, an Excel spreadsheet written by Robert Newcombe and available free from his excellent website https://www.crcpress.com/Confidence-Intervals-for-Proportions-and-Related-Measures-of-Effect-Size/Newcombe/p/book/9781439812785 (see box 2.9).

We note that there are several so-called exact methods for calculating confidence intervals for proportions and different ones will give slightly different values, but the differences will be unimportant unless the sample is very small.

6.3 Presenting the results of prevalence studies

The prevalence of chlamydial infection, 0.029, was small and so was presented as a percentage, 2.9%, rather than as a proportion as this avoids having lots of zeros and makes it easier to read (box 6.1). Some proportions of interest may be even smaller, such as cause-specific mortality, and are therefore expressed as the number of events per 1000 or even per 100,000. For example, perinatal mortality is usually expressed as the number of deaths per 1000 births and so it is best to choose this format to present the proportion.

In addition to presenting the actual prevalence and confidence interval, it is important to describe the recruitment process and the main characteristics of the sample obtained to allow the results to be interpreted in context and to make it clear which population the results can be generalized to (see sections 5.3–5.5, and 5.7).

Note that in the original paper (Oakeshott et al. 1998), the large sample Normal approximation was used (proportion ±1.96 standard errors) to calculate the 95% confidence interval and this gives a slightly different confidence interval (2.0% to 3.8%). The large sample assumption was reasonable because the numbers were large and the differences in the limits are small.

When the sample is small or there are few subjects with the condition, the exact binomial method must be used to calculate the confidence intervals; otherwise, invalid values may be obtained. A rule of thumb is that the exact method should be used if the number of subjects both with and without the condition is less than 5. If you get a confidence interval for a proportion with a negative lower limit or an upper limit above 1, this is an indication that the large sample assumptions are not met. In such cases the negative limits should not be reset to 0, or limits which exceed 1 be reset to 1, since the confidence limits will then be too narrow. Instead, the exact method should be used.

6.4 Screening and diagnostic studies: Sensitivity and specificity

These studies are used to evaluate the usefulness of a new screening technique to predict future adverse events. Sensitivity and specificity are calculated to summarize the performance of the new test compared to a 'gold standard' diagnosis.

To illustrate the presentation of sensitivity and specificity, we will use data from a sub-study of the larger UKOS study. The aim of the sub-study was to validate a parental questionnaire as a substitute for a specialist clinical assessment in children who had been born very prematurely. The parental questionnaire measured cognitive development at age 2 years, in children who had been born very prematurely, by deriving a score from information collected on the children's vocabulary, sentence complexity, and non-verbal cognition. The validation study sought to identify the particular parental questionnaire score that corresponded to a predefined point on the clinical assessment scale that was commonly

---

Box 6.1 Presenting a prevalence   *EXAMPLE*

Chlamydia infection in General Practice

Aim of the study To estimate the prevalence of chlamydial infection.

Study design Cross-sectional prevalence study.

Patient population 1382 women aged 16–34 presenting for smear tests in 30 Inner London General Practices.

Description

Methods section The prevalence and exact 95% binomial confidence interval were calculated.

Results section Forty of the 1382 women tested positive for chlamydial infection (2.9%; 95% confidence interval 2.1% to 3.9%).

For further information see Oakeshott P, Kerry S, H S, Hay P. Opportunistic screening for chlamydial infection at time of cervical smear testing in general practice: prevalence study. *BMJ* 1998; 316:351–352.

used to identify children with developmental delay. Hence, the clinical assessment was regarded as the gold standard, and the parental questionnaire as the new screening test.

6.5 **Presentation of sensitivity and specificity**

Sometimes sensitivity and specificity are given as proportions and sometimes as percentages. It does not really matter since the proportions are usually close to 1 and so there is no confusion as to which have been used. Percentages are used here.

Box 6.2 shows the presentation of the validation study of the screening tool. Figure 6.2 shows how to calculate the sensitivity and specificity in Stata. Note this was a two-stage process with the numbers obtained from the two-way table being entered manually into the program.

Note that calculation using the large sample approximation may be dubious for these data because sensitivity and specificity are likely to be close to 100% and so the approximations involved may not hold.

6.6 **Comment on results**

Figure 6.2 shows that the sensitivity and specificity in the validation study were both greater than 80% and so fairly high, indicating that the parental questionnaire performed

---

Box 6.2 Presenting sensitivity and specificity   *EXAMPLE*

UKOS validation study

Aim of study To validate a new screening tool for cognitive function in children.

Study design Cross-sectional screening study.

Patient population 64 parents and their children aged 2 years who were born very prematurely.

Description

Methods section Sensitivity and specificity were calculated with exact 95% binomial confidence intervals.

Results section Twenty-five percent of children (16/64) scored below the cut-off for normal development using the MDI clinical assessment. Thirteen of the 16 were correctly classified as developmentally delayed by the parental questionnaire, giving a sensitivity of 81% (95% CI: 54% to 96%). Of the 48 children classified as having normal development, 39 were correctly classified by the parental questionnaire giving a specificity of 81% (95% CI: 67% to 91%).

For further information see Johnson S, Marlow N, Wolke D, Davidson L, Marston L, O'Hare A et al. Validation of a parent report measure of cognitive development in very preterm infants. *Dev Med Child Neurol* 2004; 46:389–397.

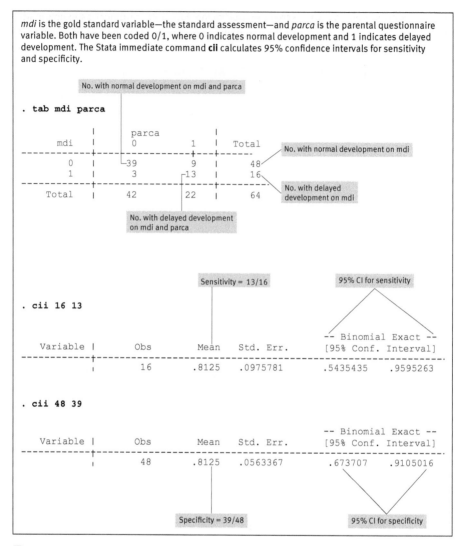

mdi is the gold standard variable—the standard assessment—and *parca* is the parental questionnaire variable. Both have been coded 0/1, where 0 indicates normal development and 1 indicates delayed development. The Stata immediate command **cii** calculates 95% confidence intervals for sensitivity and specificity.

Figure 6.2 Calculating sensitivity (Stata)

reasonably well. However, the confidence intervals were wide, especially for the sensitivity, which was based on only 16 observations.

6.7 **Screening studies for rare conditions**

It is important to give the actual numbers when presenting sensitivity and specificity, and a confidence interval is usually informative. Reporting full details allows the reader to judge the precision of the estimates; this is especially important when there are very few 'positives' and therefore the precision of the sensitivity is low.

Box 6.3 shows an example of a screening study where the total number of subjects studied was quite large (360), but where the number who were positive for various outcomes was much smaller (ranging from 3 to 43) because the outcomes were rare. Thus, despite the large overall sample size, the estimates of sensitivity were based on small numbers and

---

Box 6.3 Screening study with rare condition   *EXAMPLE*

Ultrasound study
Aim of study

To investigate the use of Doppler ultrasound in pregnancy at 23 weeks gestation to predict the development of adverse perinatal outcomes in twin pregnancies.

Study population

360 pregnant women carrying twins, who had had Doppler ultrasound examination at 22–24 weeks gestation.

Ultrasound measurements

- Pulsatility index (≥95th centile)
- Bilateral notches

Outcomes

- Pre-eclampsia
- Fetal growth retardation (FGR)
- Abruption
- Intrauterine death
- Preterm delivery ≤32 weeks

Extract of results

Sensitivity (95% CI) for pulsatility index (≥95th centile):

- Pre-eclampsia: 7/21 = 33% (15% to 57%)
- FGR in both twins: 3/31 = 10% (2% to 26%)
- Abruption: 2/3 = 67% (9% to 99%)
- Intrauterine death: 2/6 = 33% (4% to 78%)
- Delivery: ≤32 wk 8/43 = 19% (8% to 33%)

Comment

Two screening measures were tested on several outcomes. Adverse outcomes were rare so sensitivities were all based on small numbers even though the total sample size, 360, was quite large. Thus the confidence intervals were very wide showing that the estimates were imprecise.

For further information see Yu CK, Papageorghiou AT, Boli A, Cacho AM, Nicolaides KH. Screening for pre-eclampsia and fetal growth restriction in twin pregnancies at 23 weeks of gestation by transvaginal uterine artery Doppler. *Ultrasound Obstet Gynecol* 2002; 20:535–540.

> **Box 6.4 Further references to statistical details presented**
> **in this chapter**   *INFORMATION*
>
> **Confidence intervals for single proportions**
>
> Peacock and Peacock 2011 (chapter 8), Altman 1991 (chapter 10), Altman et al. 2000 (chapter 6), Bland 2015 (chapter 8), Machin et al. 2007 (chapter 6), Kirkwood and Sterne 2003 (chapter 15)
>
> **Sensitivity and specificity**
>
> Peacock and Peacock 2011 (chapter 9), Altman 1991 (chapter 14), Bland 2015 (chapter 20), Kirkwood and Sterne 2003 (chapter 36)

were imprecise. This situation is not uncommon and is another reason why it is important to include the numbers from which sensitivity and specificity was calculated, and confidence intervals, as well as the proportions themselves.

6.8 Extensions to sensitivity and specificity

Receiver operating characteristic (ROC) curves can be used to determine the best cut-off when there are several possible values. This method was used in the UKOS validation study described earlier. Details of ROC curves are omitted here but details and an example can be found in Peacock and Peacock 2011 (page 348), and in Altman and Bland 1994.

Sometimes it is useful to calculate other statistics, such as the positive predictive value and the negative predictive value. The presentation of these statistics is the same as for sensitivity and specificity as they are also essentially simple proportions (see Peacock and Peacock 2011 (chapter 9)). It is possible to compare the performance of two or more screening tools by comparing quantities like the sensitivity and specificity, and area under the ROC curve. Such analyses take account of the precision of the estimates. Details are beyond the scope of this book.

Area under the ROC curve can also be used to summarize the relationship between a dichotomous outcome and a predictor variable. This can be helpful where there are several possible predictor variables, as the areas under the ROC curves can be compared to see which factors are more closely related to the outcome. An example can be found in table 1 of the paper by May et al. 2011.

6.9 Further reading

The references given in box 6.4 provide further information on the topics in this chapter.

Box 6.5 Presenting single proportions   *CHAPTER SUMMARY*

- Give numbers of subjects as well as the proportion or percentage
- Choose an appropriate presentation for a prevalence which avoids too many zeros, e.g. percentage, or rate per 1,000, or rate per 100,000, etc.
- Sensitivity and specificity can be presented either as proportions or percentages, as the values tend to be close to 100%
- Present 95% confidence interval for prevalence/sensitivity/specificity unless the number of subjects is very small

CHAPTER 7

Comparing two groups

7.1   Introduction 72
7.2   Graphical presentation of continuous unpaired data 72
7.3   Continuous unpaired data: The two-sample *t* test 75
7.4   Mann–Whitney *U* test 79
7.5   Comparing two proportions 82
7.6   Further reading 96

7.1 Introduction

Subjects are often grouped together according to a common characteristic and then the groups compared with each other. These might be different treatment groups in a clinical trial, subjects with different exposures to a risk factor, or cases and controls in an unmatched case-control study. In a case-control study, if each case has one or more controls matched to it, then methods for analysing matched data should be used as described in chapter 8. In this chapter we consider three different situations: comparing two groups using a *t* test, comparing two groups using a Mann—Whitney *U* test, and comparing two proportions. Chapter 11 describes how to compare survival curves in two or more groups.

7.2 Graphical presentation of continuous unpaired data

In many situations it is sufficient to describe the data using summary statistics such as the mean and standard deviation, or median and range. Sometimes the distribution is of interest and a graphical presentation that allows the two groups to be compared is useful. This is illustrated here by two examples from the same study, in which twelve villages in Ghana took part in a health education trial to reduce salt intake (Kerry et al. 2005a). Blood pressure and body mass index were measured, before the intervention began, for 338 women living in six semi-urban villages, compared to 290 women living in six rural villages.

There are several ways to present continuous data graphically, and the choice is largely a personal one. Figure 7.1 presents two separate histograms, and figure 7.2 presents overlapping density plots for the same data. Both figures show that body mass index is higher in the semi-urban women, with a long tail at the upper end of the distribution. Body mass index is still skewed in the rural areas but less so, and

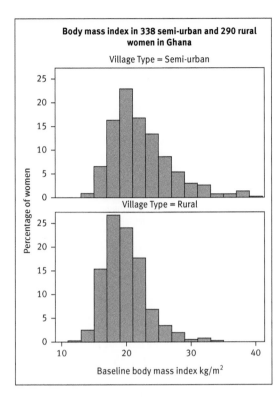

📑 **Figure 7.1** Histograms of two groups on one graph (SAS)

For further information see Kerry SM, Micah FB, Plange-Rhule J, Eastwood JB, Cappuccio FP. Blood pressure and body mass index in lean rural and semi-urban subjects in West Africa. *J Hypertens* 2005(a); 23:1645–1651.

a greater proportion of rural women are underweight (as defined by a body mass index below 18 kg/m²).

Alternatively, a box and whisker plot can be drawn as shown in figure 7.3. The horizontal line in the middle of each box indicates the median of each group, while the top and bottom horizontal lines indicate the upper and lower quartiles, respectively, and so the length of the box is the interquartile range (IQR). The diamond indicates the mean in this SAS plot but note that Stata, SPSS, and R do not mark the mean. Extreme values or outliers

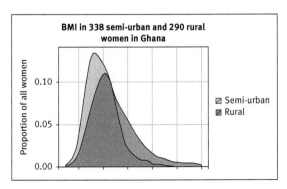

📑 **Figure 7.2** Overlapping density plots for two groups (R)

For further information see Kerry SM, Micah FB, Plange-Rhule J, Eastwood JB, Cappuccio FP. Blood pressure and body mass index in lean rural and semi-urban subjects in West Africa. *J Hypertens* 2005(a); 23:1645–1651.

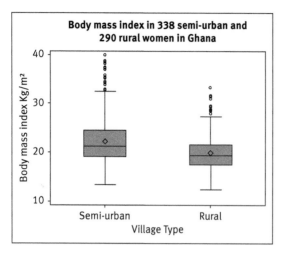

⬚ **Figure 7.3** Box and whisker plot for a continuous variable in two groups (SAS)

For further information see Kerry SM, Micah FB, Plange-Rhule J, Eastwood JB, Cappuccio FP. Blood pressure and body mass index in lean rural and semi-urban subjects in West Africa. *J Hypertens* 2005(a); 23:1645–1651.

are indicated as separate points. In this figure, extreme values are only seen at the top end of the distribution, as it is positively skewed, and all the observations at the lower end fall within the range expected. In SAS, Stata, R, and SPSS, outliers are defined as observations that are more extreme than 1.5 × IQR from either quartile. The box plot shows similar features to the histograms in figures 7.1 to 7.2. A further possibility is the use of a violin plot to demonstrate the two distributions (figure 7.4).

The numbers of women in these samples were large, leading to fairly smooth graphs. With small datasets, where a histogram, plot, or graph may be uneven, a dot plot of the data may be more useful. To illustrate this we use the percentage of villagers who had electricity in their homes in each of the twelve villages in the Ghana study. This is shown in figure 7.5 (Kerry et al. 2005a).

There were six villages in each group, and two of the rural villages had no electricity at all. Note that the points have been 'jittered' using a technique which adds a small amount

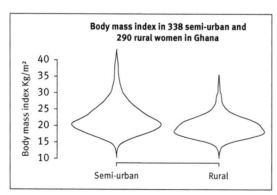

⬚ **Figure 7.4** Violin plot for a continuous variable comparing two groups (R)

For further information see Kerry SM, Micah FB, Plange-Rhule J, Eastwood JB, Cappuccio FP. Blood pressure and body mass index in lean rural and semi-urban subjects in West Africa. *J Hypertens* 2005(a); 23:1645–1651.

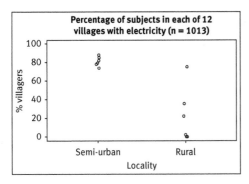

Figure 7.5 Dot plot for a continuous variable comparing two groups (R)

For further information see Kerry SM, Micah FB, Plange-Rhule J, Eastwood JB, Cappuccio FP. Blood pressure and body mass index in lean rural and semi-urban subjects in West Africa. *J Hypertens* 2005(a); 23:1645–1651.

of random variability to the placing of the points so that multiple points with the same value can still be seen. The graph shows that in semi-urban villages around 80% of the respondents had electricity and there was little variability between the villages. On the other hand, in rural villages there were far fewer homes with electricity but a much greater difference between villages.

7.2.1 Graphical presentation of more than two groups

The box and whisker plot and dot plot could easily be extended to more than two groups. In figure 7.3, which shows body mass index data for women, body mass index for men in semi-urban and rural areas could also be shown on the same axes.

7.3 Continuous unpaired data: The two-sample *t* test

One hundred and ten patients with peripheral vascular disease were recruited to a cohort study to investigate the predictors of mortality (Missouris et al. 2004). The analysis used a *t* test to compare the mean blood pressure at recruitment in those who subsequently died, with those who survived. Before carrying out a *t* test it is important to check that the assumptions of the *t* test hold (see box 7.1).

If the assumptions do not hold then we may fail to detect a real difference or have confidence intervals which are too wide. The histogram (figure 7.6) shows that systolic blood pressure is very slightly skewed but not enough to invalidate the *t* test. For a full discussion of the *t* test and its assumptions see Bland 2015 (chapter 10). If the assumptions do not hold then a transformation might be considered (section 7.3.2) or a Mann—Whitney *U* rank test used (section 7.4).

7.3.1 Presenting the results of a *t* test

Since the *t* test tests the hypothesis that two population means are the same, the sample mean and the standard deviation are the most appropriate descriptive statistics to report, along with the difference in means and its 95% confidence interval. The use of the standard deviation rather than the standard error for the two groups allows the assumptions of equal variance (i.e. equal standard deviations) to be assessed by the reader. Showing the means

---

Box 7.1 The two-sample *t* test   *INFORMATION*

The *t* test is a test of significance which gives an estimate and a confidence interval as well as a *P* value

Null hypothesis Difference between the two population means is zero.

Most suitable for Continuous variables but can also be used for scores.

Assumptions Data are Normally distributed in both groups and standard deviations of the two groups are the same.

Deviations from the assumptions The *t* test can be used when:

* Data are symmetric even if non-Normal
* Data are symmetric but display digit preference
* Two samples are the same size even if data are moderately skewed
* Data are highly skewed but the groups are large (>50 in each group)

Checking the assumptions

* Does a histogram of the data in each group look symmetric? Note that small samples will often display an uneven distribution which can be ignored
* Are the SDs similar? If the SD is bigger in the group with the biggest mean this may indicate skewness
* If data are skewed, try to transform, otherwise power is lost

Unequal variances

* Often an indication of skewness
* Consider using modified *t* test; such Satterthwaite's test, available in Stata, SAS, R, and SPSS

Levene's test for equality of variance

* Routinely given by SPSS but it is of limited value
* When samples are small, the test may not pick up important differences
* When samples are large, the test may pick up differences which will not affect the results of the *t* test

---

of the two groups helps to describe the patient groups and is also a check on the direction of the difference in means.

The results of the two-sample *t* test are shown in figure 7.7. Box 7.2 gives an illustration of how to present these findings. The analysis shows that mean systolic and diastolic blood pressure at recruitment was 4 mm Hg higher in those who died compared to those who survived, but the difference is not statistically significant. Note that SPSS gives two versions of the results for the *t* test, (i) assuming equal variances and (ii) assuming unequal variances. Other packages, such as Stata, give only the test assuming equal variances by default.

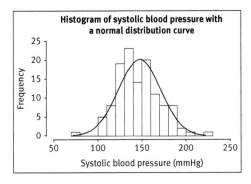

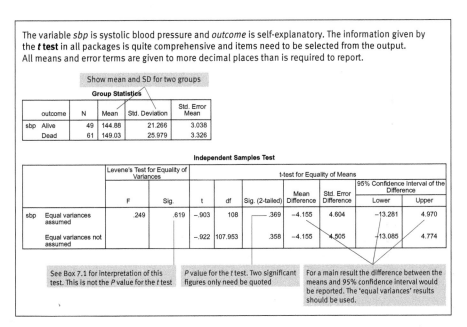

🕮 **Figure 7.6** Histogram of a variable to check for Normality (R)

In this example the difference is trivial but power will be lost if incorrect assumptions are made (see box 7.1).

7.3.2 Logarithmic transformations

Figure 7.8 shows histograms for a skewed variable, serum creatinine level, before and after logarithmic (log) transformation. The data are still slightly skewed after log transformation but, since the groups are fairly equal in size and both quite large, the slight skewness should not affect the *t* test (see Bland 2015 (chapter 10) for a fuller discussion). The results of these descriptive analyses would not normally be reported in the main body of a report,

The variable *sbp* is systolic blood pressure and *outcome* is self-explanatory. The information given by the ***t* test** in all packages is quite comprehensive and items need to be selected from the output. All means and error terms are given to more decimal places than is required to report.

Show mean and SD for two groups

Group Statistics

outcome		N	Mean	Std. Deviation	Std. Error Mean
sbp	Alive	49	144.88	21.266	3.038
	Dead	61	149.03	25.979	3.326

Independent Samples Test

		Levene's Test for Equality of Variances		t-test for Equality of Means					95% Confidence Interval of the Difference	
		F	Sig.	t	df	Sig. (2-tailed)	Mean Difference	Std. Error Difference	Lower	Upper
sbp	Equal variances assumed	.249	.619	−.903	108	.369	−4.155	4.604	−13.281	4.970
	Equal variances not assumed			−.922	107.953	.358	−4.155	4.505	−13.085	4.774

See Box 7.1 for interpretation of this test. This is not the *P* value for the *t* test

P value for the *t* test. Two significant figures only need be quoted

For a main result the difference between the means and 95% confidence interval would be reported. The 'equal variances' results should be used.

🕮 **Figure 7.7** Output for an unpaired *t* test (SPSS)

Box 7.2 Presenting the results of a *t* test   *EXAMPLE*

Peripheral Vascular Disease study

Aim of study To assess the long-term survival of patients with peripheral vascular disease (PVD) and to investigate the impact of the presence of risk factors on mortality.

Study design Cohort study.

Patient population Consecutive patients with peripheral vascular disease, who were referred for angiography and found to have angiographic evidence of PVD.

Aim of analysis To compare baseline blood pressure in survivors and those who died.

Table **Comparison of blood pressure in survivors and those who died.**

	Mean (SD)		Difference (95% CI)	P value
	Died (N=61)	**Survived (N=49)**		
Systolic blood pressure (mmHg)	149 (26)	145 (21)	4 (−5 to 13)	0.37
Diastolic blood pressure (mmHg)	78 (14)	74 (10)	4 (−1 to 9)	0.085

Description

Methods section Mean blood pressure values between patients who died and who survived were compared using unpaired *t* tests.

Results section Mean blood pressure values were 4 mmHg higher in those who died than those who survived but this difference was not statistically significant.

For further information see Missouris CG, Kalaitzidis RG, Kerry SM, Cappuccio FP. Predictors of mortality on patients with peripheral vascular disease: a prospective follow- up study. *Br J Diabetes Vasc Dis* 2004; 4:196–200.

---

particularly if space is limited (as in a journal paper), unless the distribution of the variable was of prime interest.

It is worth noting that transforming the data using logarithms will not be suitable for all skewed data and that transformation changes the hypothesis being tested (box 7.3).

The results of the *t* test are shown in figure 7.9. Back-transformation, with a calculator or spreadsheet/program, is required to obtain the ratio of the geometric means and 95% confidence intervals. Since only the 95% confidence intervals can be back-transformed to give sensible results, we suggest 95% confidence intervals are used throughout, as in box 7.4.

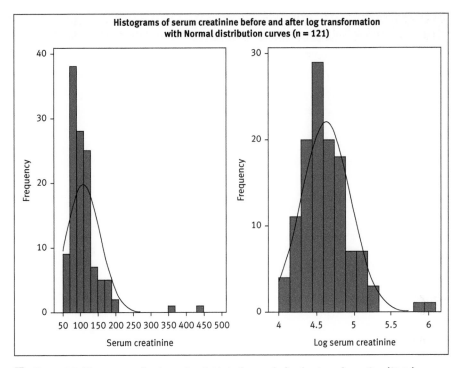

Figure 7.8 Histograms of a skewed variable before and after log transformation (Stata)

7.3.3 Further analysis of the data

Sometimes we may wish to investigate whether the differences between the means (or the lack of difference) is due to a third factor. One way of doing this is by multiple regression analysis. Mathematically, multiple regression analysis is an extension of the *t* test and has similar assumptions. If we use multiple regression analysis, we can then present the difference in means alongside the difference in means after adjusting for the third factor. We show how to do this and present these analyses in chapter 10.

7.4 **Mann–Whitney *U* test**

The Mann–Whitney *U* test is a test based on the ranks of the data. It is equivalent to the Wilcoxon two-sample test, and both compare two independent groups. The Mann—Whitney *U* test can be used where there is no suitable Normalizing transformation or where the data are in the form of a score (box 7.5). This test is illustrated here by comparing the number of portions of fruit and vegetables per day eaten by smokers and non-smokers. The data come from the baseline questionnaire of subjects enrolled into a trial of an intervention to increase the consumption of fruit and

---

Box 7.3 The _t_ test on log transformed data   _INFORMATION_

Null hypothesis The ratio of the population geometric means equals 1.

Used for Continuous variables with positive skewness and positive values.

Assumptions Apply to log transformed data: transformed data are Normally distributed and standard deviations of the two groups are the same.

Not suitable for
- Highly skewed data as log transformation will not give Normal distribution, e.g. assay results where many subjects have undetectable levels
- Cost data where the main interest is usually in the arithmetic mean which relates directly to cost per patient

Note
- Data with a small number of zero values can be log transformed by adding a small constant to the zero values before transformation. If there are many zeros, the data will be highly skewed and this transformation will not work. For other options in such cases see Bland and Peacock 2000 (chapter 10).
- Bootstrapping methods can be used to overcome problems with skewed cost data or, if the dataset is large enough, a nice solution is to fit a generalized linear model that provides means but allows for the non-Normal error structure (see Barber and Thompson 2004)

---

vegetables among low-income families (Eat for Life study, Steptoe et al. 2003). The data are tabulated in figure 7.10.

As the Mann–Whitney *U* test is based on ranks, the median (middle rank) and inter-quartile range are the most appropriate summary statistics to report; however, the test does not provide a 95% confidence interval, only a *P* value.

Figure 7.10 shows the output for the data, and box 7.6 shows how the results can be presented. Median and interquartile ranges have been used to present the fruit and vegetable consumption in the two groups.

In situations where there are only a small number of possible values and many equal values (ties) in the data, the medians in two groups may be the same even if there is a tendency for one group to have higher values than the other group. In this case it may be more informative to give the percentage below a chosen cut point. In the Eat for Life study, 69% of non-smokers and 90% of smokers consumed less than 5 portions of fruit and vegetables per day. Public health campaigns have promoted eating 5 portions per day so this would seem a good cut point to use if additional summary data were needed.

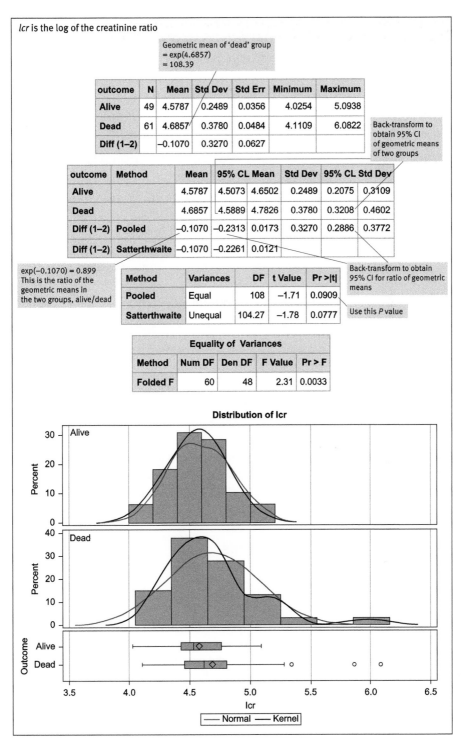

lcr is the log of the creatinine ratio

Geometric mean of 'dead' group
= exp(4.6857)
= 108.39

outcome	N	Mean	Std Dev	Std Err	Minimum	Maximum
Alive	49	4.5787	0.2489	0.0356	4.0254	5.0938
Dead	61	4.6857	0.3780	0.0484	4.1109	6.0822
Diff (1–2)		−0.1070	0.3270	0.0627		

Back-transform to obtain 95% CI of geometric means of two groups

outcome	Method	Mean	95% CL Mean	Std Dev	95% CL Std Dev
Alive		4.5787	4.5073 4.6502	0.2489	0.2075 0.3109
Dead		4.6857	4.5889 4.7826	0.3780	0.3208 0.4602
Diff (1–2)	Pooled	−0.1070	−0.2313 0.0173	0.3270	0.2886 0.3772
Diff (1–2)	Satterthwaite	−0.1070	−0.2261 0.0121		

exp(−0.1070) = 0.899
This is the ratio of the geometric means in the two groups, alive/dead

Back-transform to obtain 95% CI for ratio of geometric means

Method	Variances	DF	t Value	Pr >|t|
Pooled	Equal	108	−1.71	0.0909
Satterthwaite	Unequal	104.27	−1.78	0.0777

Use this *P* value

Equality of Variances				
Method	Num DF	Den DF	F Value	Pr > F
Folded F	60	48	2.31	0.0033

Distribution of lcr

Figure 7.9 Output for back-transforming the *t* test data (SAS)

Box 7.4 Presenting the findings of a *t* test on log transformed data   *EXAMPLE*

Peripheral Vascular Disease study

Aim of study To assess the long-term survival of patients with peripheral vascular disease (PVD) and to investigate the impact of the presence of risk factors on mortality.

Study design Cohort study.

Patient population Consecutive patients with PVD who were referred for angiography and found to have angiographic evidence of PVD.

Aim of analysis To compare baseline serum creatinine in survivors and those who died.

Table **Comparison of serum creatinine in survivors and those who died.**

	Geometric mean (95% CI)		Ratio of geometric means (survived/died)	
	Died (N=61)	Survived (N=49)	(95% CI)	P value
Serum creatinine at baseline (mmol/l)	108 (98, 119)	97 (91, 105)	0.90 (0.79, 1.02)	0.091

Description

Methods section Serum creatinine values were positively skewed and so the raw data were log-transformed prior to using *t* test. The results are presented as geometric means and the ratio of geometric means with 95% confidence intervals.

Results section Mean serum creatinine values were 10% lower in those who survived than in those who died but this difference was not statistically significant.

For further information see Missouris CG, Kalaitzidis RG, Kerry SM, Cappuccio FP. Predictors of mortality on patients with peripheral vascular disease: a prospective follow- up study. *Br J Diabetes Vasc Dis* 2004; 4:196–200.

7.5 Comparing two proportions

7.5.1 The chi-squared test

The simplest test of two proportions is the chi-squared test, often written χ^2. The main uses and assumptions of the test are given in box 7.7.

The chi-squared test is often used for analysing surveys where the response to various questions is cross-classified by other variables. For example, a student questionnaire on obesity investigated nutrition and exercise in the students' families and friends. This questionnaire was produced by the students in class and each student collected data from two friends or family members, thus giving a reasonable total sample size when all data were pooled. (The survey was used as a teaching tool and is

| Box 7.5 Mann–Whitney *U* test | *INFORMATION* |

Null hypothesis Observations from one group do not tend to have higher or lower ranking than those from the other group.

Most suitable for
- Scores
- Continuous variables that cannot be transformed to a Normal distribution

Assumptions Data can be ranked.

Not suitable for Cost data where the main interest is usually in the arithmetic mean, which relates directly to cost per patient.

Limitations
- Needs more than three observations in each group for statistical significance to be possible if using $P = 0.05$, and more for lower significance level
- Significance test only

Cautionary note This does not test the hypothesis that the medians are the same unless we make very strong assumptions. It is possible for one group to have higher ranks than the other overall, but to have the same median, particularly where there are a lot of ties.

Notes
- Gives same *P* value as Wilcoxon unpaired test
- Analogue of two-sample *t* test

therefore not perfect! However, the data are useful for illustrating the presentation of a simple survey.)

7.5.2 Presenting chi-squared tests

When presenting the results of chi-squared tests new researchers sometimes present each chi-squared test as a separate table, therefore including unnecessary information given by computer programs. This makes it hard to absorb the findings and also makes the results section very long. In box 7.8 we show how several chi-squared tests can be presented concisely in one table. Note that, where the outcome is dichotomous, it is unnecessary to give the proportion who respond negatively to the questions as well as the proportion who respond positively, since one can easily be deduced from the other. For example, we do not need to give the proportion who take no exercise as well as the proportion who do take exercise.

We do not report the actual chi-squared test statistic since we do not think it necessary if the data are given. We do not calculate confidence intervals since the survey was purely descriptive and confidence intervals would not provide any useful additional information here. Later on in this chapter we give examples where estimates and confidence intervals should be included. Examples given in this chapter show how to extract the relevant information from computer output for the chi-squared test (figure 7.11).

(a)

smokeas is coded 0 for non-smokers and 1 for smokers. frandveg is the number of portions of fruit and vegetables eaten per day.

```
. tabulate frandveg smokeas

                    smokeas
   frandveg      0           1         Total

          0      0           1             1
         .5      1           0             1
          1      7           7            14
        1.5      5           1             6
          2     33          21            54
        2.5     12           4            16
          3     28          26            54
        3.5      4           3             7
          4     26          19            45
        4.5      8           0             8
          5     18           3            21
        5.5      3           0             3
          6     16           3            19
          7      9           2            11
        7.5      1           0             1
          8      5           0             5
          9      1           1             2
         10      1           0             1
         11      1           0             1
         13      1           0             1

      Total    180          91           271
```

(b)

```
. ranksum frandveg, by (smokeas)


Two-sample Wilcoxon rank-sum (Mann-Whitney) test

     smokeas │     obs     rank sum     expected

           0 │     180        26342        24480
           1 │      91        10514        12376

    combined │     271        36856        36856

unadjusted variance      371280.00
adjustment for ties       -8046.17

adjusted variance        363233.83

Ho: frandveg (smokeas==0) = frandveg (smokeas==1)
             z = 3.089
    Prob > |z| = 0.0020
```

P value for Mann–Whitney U test

📖 **Figure 7.10** (a) Table for data prior to using Mann–Whitney U test (Stata) (b) Output for Mann–Whitney U test (Stata)

Box 7.6 Presenting results of a Mann–Whitney *U* test   *EXAMPLE*

Eat for Life study

Aim of the study To see if a behavioural intervention can increase fruit and vegetable consumption in low-income families.

Study design Randomized controlled trial.

Patient population Patients recruited from one General Practice age/sex register.

Aim of the analysis To compare fruit and vegetable consumption in smokers and non-smokers.

Description

Methods section The fruit and vegetable scores from smokers and non-smokers were compared using a Mann–Whitney *U* test. The data are presented as medians and interquartile range (IQR).

Results section The median (IQR) number of portions of fruit and vegetable eaten per day at baseline among smokers was 3 (2, 4) and 3.75 (2, 5) among non-smokers. Smokers reported significantly lower consumption than non-smokers ($P = 0.002$).

For further information see Steptoe A, Perkins-Porras L, McKay C, Rink E, Hilton S, Cappuccio FP. Behavioural counselling to increase consumption of fruit and vegetables in low income adults: randomised trial. *BMJ* 2003; 326:855–860.

Note that the 2×2 chi-squared test assumes that the sample is 'large' and will be invalid in small samples. A rule of thumb that is widely used to define a 'large' sample is one in which all the chi-squared test expected values are greater than 5. The chi-squared test with the continuity correction is better than the ordinary chi-squared test in small sample situations or, alternatively, Fisher's exact test can be used. In a large sample, both Fisher's exact and the chi-squared test will give similar P values and should therefore lead to the same conclusions.

Box 7.7 The chi-squared test for two proportions   *INFORMATION*

Null hypothesis The proportion of individuals in the population with the characteristic is the same in the two groups.

Suitable for Variables where subjects fall into one of two categories.

Assumptions Large sample test. All expected values must be greater than 5.

Limitations Significance test only, consider using risk difference, relative risk, or odds ratio to assess size of the difference between the groups.

Box 7.8 Presenting the results of survey data with several chi-squared tests *EXAMPLE*

Obesity study

Aim of the study To investigate nutrition, exercise, and attitudes to obesity in men and women.

Participants Family and friends of students.

Aim of the analysis To see if reported nutrition, exercise, and attitudes to obesity differed in men and women.

Description

Methods section The differences in the proportions of men and women responding positively to each question were tested using the chi-squared test. Results are presented as percentages and the corresponding *P* value.

Results section

Table **Nutrition, exercise, and attitudes to obesity in men and women**

Question/opinion	Men	Women	P value
	N=34	**N=47**	
Eats a healthy diet	79% (27/34)	77% (36/47)	0.76
Eats fatty food weekly or more	29% (10/34)	36% (17/47)	0.52
Eats vegetables daily	65% (22/34)	66% (31/47)	0.91
Takes some exercise	71% (24/34)	64% (30/47)	0.52
Obesity is person's own business	64% (21/33)	42% (19/45)	0.062
Obesity is a medical issue for NHS	27% (9/33)	49% (22/45)	0.054

Eighty-one questionnaires were returned, 34 from men and 47 from women. Most respondents reported eating a healthy diet, and the majority eat vegetables every day, eat fatty foods infrequently, and take some exercise. The percentages were similar in men and women. More men than women thought that obesity was a personal affair, and more women than men thought that obesity was an issue for the NHS to deal with. The differences between men and women in these attitude questions were of borderline statistical significance.

7.5.3 The chi-squared test and estimates of effect

The main drawback of the chi-squared test is that it is a test of significance only; it does not tell us how large the difference between the groups is. There are three main ways to compare proportions: to calculate the difference in the proportions; to calculate the ratio of the proportions; and to calculate the ratio of the odds. These different estimates are summarized in box 7.9. The choice of whether to use a difference or a ratio of proportions *bv* is the binary variable denoting bacterial vaginosis. **tabulate** is useful as it keeps the value labels instead of using 'exposed' and unexposed' and 'cases' and 'controls' (non-cases). However, **cs** provides the risk of bv in each group plus the relative risk and risk difference with 95% confidence intervals. Usually either relative risk or risk difference is reported. For **cs** to give correct relative risk, variables must be coded as 0/1 where 0 = absence of risk factor, 1 = presence of risk factor; 0 = control and 1 = case.

. **tabulate bv age, col chi2**

```
Key

    frequency
  column percentage
```

	agegrp		
bv	>=25	<25	Total
No	911	116	1,027
	86.68	77.33	85.51
Yes	140	34	174
	13.32	22.67	14.49
Total	1,051	150	1,201
	100.00	100.00	100.00

> **tabulate** (can be shortened to **tab**) gives percentage of bv positive in the 'under 25' group while **cs** gives the proportion

Pearson chi2(1) =   9.2549   Pr = 0.002

> P value for chi-squared test. If small samples use Fisher's exact test

. **cs bv age**

	agegrp		
	Exposed	Unexposed	Total
Cases	34	140	174
Noncases	116	911	1027
Total	150	1051	1201
Risk	.2266667	.1332065	.1448793
	Point estimate		[95% Conf. Interval]
Risk difference	.0934602		.0233808 .1635396
Risk ratio	1.701619		1.219177 2.374969
Attr. frac. ex.	.4123244		.1797746 .5789418
Attr. frac. pop	.0805691		

chi2(1) = 9.25   Pr>chi2 = 0.0023

> Risk difference with 95% confidence interval 0.2267 − 0.1332 = 0.0935

> Relative risk (risk ratio) and its 95% confidence interval. It is the ratio of the risks in each group 0.2267/0.1332 = 1.70

Cautionary note: Unlike SPSS and SAS, Stata and some R packages will not give a warning when the numbers in each cell are too small for the test to be valid. See Box 7.7 for guidelines.

Figure 7.11 Output for chi-squared test, relative risk, and risk difference (Stata)

> **Box 7.9 Which estimate to use for comparing proportions?**   *HELPFUL TIPS*
>
> We will call the two proportions p_1 and p_2.
>
> *Risk difference: $p_1 - p_2$*
> - Most straightforward estimate and useful for surveys
> - Use if actual size of difference is of interest
> - Can be useful for randomized trials as relates to the number needed to treat (1/risk difference)
>
> *Relative risk: p_1/p_2*
> - Use if the relative difference is of interest
> - Useful when comparing the size of effect for several factors
> - Easier to interpret than the odds ratio
> - Adjust for other factors using Poisson regression, but this can be problematic when outcome is common
> - Do not use for case-control studies
>
> *Odds ratio: ad/bc where a, b, c, d are frequencies in 2 × 2 table*
> - Approximates to relative risk if outcome is rare
> - Can be misinterpreted where outcome is common
> - Use for case-control studies
> - Easier to adjust for other factors than relative risks
> - Adjust for other factors using logistic regression

depends partly on the context and partly on personal preference (see box 7.9 for our suggestions).

7.5.4 Relative risk

In the Early Pregnancy study, the risk of bacterial vaginosis could be calculated for all women, and in women with and without various risk factors (Oakeshott et al. 2002). Table 5.1 shows the risk of bacterial vaginosis in women aged less than 25, and women aged 25 years or more. They are compared using a relative risk. Figure 7.11 shows the analyses to calculate the relative risk. Box 7.10 shows how to present these results within the text. (The same data are also shown in tables 5.1 and 5.2, and figure 5.2.)

From any two-way table it is possible to obtain eight different values for a risk ratio, so it is important to code the variables appropriately in order to obtain the right one. Figure 7.11 shows the coding used to produce the correct results. It is fairly simple to check the relative risk by hand by dividing one proportion by the other on a calculator. We recommend doing this as a way of checking that the program is producing the expected relative risk estimate. A useful alternative to using the program to calculate confidence intervals for the relative risk is to use ODDSRATIOANDRR, an Excel spreadsheet available from https://www.crcpress.com/Confidence-Intervals-for-Proportions-and-Related-Measures-of-Effect-Size/Newcombe/p/book/9781439812785.

Box 7.10 Presenting the results of relative risk   *EXAMPLE*

Early Pregnancy study

Aim of the study To see if miscarriage is associated with bacterial vaginosis.

Study design Cohort study.

Patient population Women booking for antenatal care with General Practitioner.

Aim of the analysis To investigate risk factors for bacterial vaginosis.

Description

Methods section The risk of bacterial vaginosis in women with and without each risk factor is presented and the relative risk used to assess the association of the infection with each risk factor, along with the 95% confidence interval.

Results section The prevalence of bacterial vaginosis was 23% in women under 25 and 13% in women 25 and over: relative risk 1.7 (1.2 to 2.4), $P = 0.002$.

Note Table 5.1 shows how the results of several risk factors can be presented in one table.

For further information see Oakeshott P, Hay P, Hay S, Steinke F, Rink E, Thomas B et al. Detection of Chlamydia trachomatis infection in early pregnancy using self-administered vaginal swabs and first pass urines: a cross-sectional community-based survey. *Br J Gen Pract* 2002; 52:830–832.

Note that different statistical programs may require different coding of the exposure variables to get the correct relative risks. For example, Stata expects that exposure is coded 0/1 for 'no'/'yes' and 0/1 for 'control'/'case', whereas in the same dataset, while 'control'/'case' is coded 0/1, exposure will need to be coded 2/1 for 'no'/'yes' to give the same relative risk estimates in SPSS. Hence, it is worth checking that the results are the right way round.

7.5.5 Odds ratio

We illustrate the calculation and presentation of an odds ratio using data from a study of sleepiness in car drivers and car crashes (Road Crash study, Connor et al. 2002). Five hundred and seventy-one car drivers involved in crashes where at least one occupant was admitted to hospital or killed (injury crash) were compared to 588 'control' car drivers. These controls were recruited while driving on public roads, and were considered to be representative of all time spent driving in the study region during the study period. Several variables were analysed but here we compare the number of drivers who had had less than 5 hours sleep in the 24 hours prior to the crash or interview.

This study was a case-control design where the sample was chosen to have approximately the same numbers of drivers who were involved in a crash (cases) as those who had not (controls). Hence, these data cannot be used to estimate the risk of a crash. Packages may have particular commands to obtain the odds ratio from a cross-tabulation (Stata) or may give both (SAS, SPSS). Hence, the user may need to choose the correct estimate to use (e.g. here the odds ratio for a case-control study).

Figure 7.12 shows the analysis results for these data, and box 7.11 shows how these results may be presented. The odds of being involved in a car crash after less than 5 hours sleep are more than twice the odds when the driver has had 5 hours sleep or more: OR 2.59 95% CI (1.65 to 4.06) $P < 0.0001$. Note that the confidence limits

Frequency Row Pct	Table of sleep by casecontrol		
sleep (length of sleep)	casecontrol (casecontrol)		
	Crashed	Safe	Total
<=5 Hours	65	30	95
	68.42	31.58	
>5 Hours	464	554	1018
	45.58	54.42	
Total	529	584	1113

Statistics for Table of sleep by casecontrol

Statistics	DF	Value	Prob	
Chi-Square	1	18.1780	<.0001	— *P* value for chi-squared test
Likelihood Ratio Chi-Square	1	18.4517	<.0001	
Continuity Adj. Chi-Square	1	17.2737	<.0001	
Mantel-Haenszel Chi-Square	1	18.1617	<.0001	
Phi Coefficient		0.1278		
Contingency Coefficient		0.1268		
Cramer's V		0.1278		

Fisher's Exact Test	
Cell (1,1) Frequency (F)	65
Left-sided Pr <= F	1.0000
Left-sided Pr >= F	<.0001
Table Probability (P)	<.0001
Two-sided Pr <= P	<.0001

Estimates of the Relative Risk (Row1/Row2)			
Type of Study	Value	95% Confidence Limits	
Case-Control (Odds Ratio)	2.5869	1.6498	4.0565
Cohort (Col1 Risk)	1.5011	1.2892	1.7479
Cohort (Col2 Risk)	0.5803	0.4293	0.7843

This row: odds ratio and 95% confidence interval

Figure 7.12 Output for the odds ratio (SAS)

Box 7.11 Presenting the results of an odds ratio   *EXAMPLE*

Road Crash study

Aim of the study To investigate risk factors for road crashes.

Study design Case-control study.

Cases Drivers who had been involved in roads crashes.

Controls Drivers who had not been involved in road crashes, recruited while driving on public roads.

Description

Methods section Odds ratios and 95% confidence intervals were calculated to assess the relationship between each risk factor and the risk of being involved in a road traffic crash.

Results section Of the 529 drivers who had been involved in a road traffic crash, 65 (12%) had had less than 5 hours sleep in the previous 24 hours, compared with 30 out of 584 who had not been vinvolved in a crash. Drivers who had had less than 5 hours sleep were more than twice as likely to be involved in a road traffic crash as those who have had more than 5 hours sleep. Odds ratio 2.59 (1.65 to 4.06), $P < 0.0001$.

Note The interpretation of the odds ratio given above assumes that road traffic crashes are relatively rare and that the odds ratio approximates to the relative risk.

For further information see Connor J, Norton R, Ameratunga S, Robinson E, Civil I, Dunn R et al. Driver sleepiness and risk of serious injury to car occupants: population based case control study. *BMJ* 2002; 324:1125.

---

produced by different packages may be slightly different due to different approximations being used.

7.5.6 Extensions to the two-proportion chi-squared test

The chi-squared test for trend is used to look for a trend in ordered proportions. In presenting such data the same principles apply as for presenting a comparison of two proportions. It may be appropriate to give the proportions in each category or to use one category as the reference and to show the relative risk or odds ratio for each of the others. Table 7.1 gives an example of how to present such data. These data are from the Birthweight study and this analysis is investigating the trend in the proportion of women with early pregnancy nausea according to the amount smoked.

In table 7.1 we give the actual chi-squared test statistic and the degrees of freedom. We recommend doing this for a trend test in order to distinguish the result from an ordinary chi-squared test on the 2 × 3 table.

As we discussed before, with a simple two-proportion situation (box 7.9) the choice of which estimates to present depends on the context and personal preference. Confidence

Table 7.1 Presenting ordered proportions   *EXAMPLE*

Birthweight study: Nausea in early pregnancy and smoking in 1511 women

Smoking category	% (no.) with nausea
Non-smoker	83% (845/1021)
Light smoker	73% (246/336)
Heavy smoker	70% (108/154)

Test for trend, $\chi^2 = 21.65$, $P < 0.0001$, DF = 1

For further information see: Meyer LC, Peacock JL, Bland JM, Anderson HR. Symptoms and health problems in pregnancy: their association with social factors, smoking, alcohol, caffeine and attitude to pregnancy. *Paediatr Perinat Epidemiol* 1994; 8:145–155.

intervals could also be added. The nausea data are further analysed, with another factor, using logistic regression later in the book (box 10.14).

The chi-squared test can also be used on two-way tables with more than two rows and columns. The presentation of the data can then either be in proportions (or percentages), calculated either across rows (i.e. so that the row proportion total is 1.0) or down the columns (so the column proportion total is 1.0). The choice of using row or column proportions depends on the context. The overall chi-squared test result can then be given. Further analyses may be done on parts of the table, if and only if the overall chi-squared test is statistically significant.

Note that all chi-squared tests are large-sample tests with the rule of thumb that at least 80% of expected values must be greater than 5 and none are less than 1 for the test to be valid. If the sample is too small then the table may be collapsed by combining rows and/or columns in an appropriate way. Alternatively, Fisher's exact test can be used.

7.5.7 Dichotomizing continuous outcomes to give proportions

Proportions occur naturally such as the proportion of babies who are boys. Proportions can also be computed 'artificially' from measurements by dichotomization. For example a patient's blood pressure may be classified as 'high' if their systolic blood pressure is 140 mmHg or more and classified as 'normal' otherwise. Dichotomizing continuous outcomes is commonly done but is problematic statistically because information is discarded and hence statistical power is lost. This means that when we dichotomize continuous data, real differences may be missed. Box 7.12 gives summary information on why dichotomization is used and why it is problematic.

Sometimes data are dichotomized and presented alongside the original data summarized as means. Box 7.12 briefly describes a statistical method that allows this to be done without the loss of statistical power, and figure 7.13 shows an example of its use in practice. In the example, children who were randomized into the UKOS study at birth were followed up again as adolescents and their lung function was measured to see if the type of ventilation used at birth was related to their lung function at age 11–14 years. The data

Box 7.12 Dichotomizing continuous outcomes   *INFORMATION*

What do we mean by dichotomization of outcomes?

- A measurement made on an individual is translated into a yes/no outcome according to whether the measurement is above or below a pre-specified cut point
- Continuous outcomes are usually summarized vusing means and standard deviations but dichotomized outcomes are summarized by the proportion above or below the cut point
- Groups are typically compared using a *t* test for means, or a chi-squared test for proportions

Why researchers dichotomize continuous outcomes

- Differences between the means in two groups can be difficult to interpret: for example, the difference in mean babies' birthweight according to mothers' smoking in pregnancy is approximately 200 g. This is difficult to interpret clinically.
- Measurements may be used to guide decisions: for example, when deciding to treat a patient for hypertension if systolic blood pressure is 140 mmHg or more.
- Measurements may be used to indicate individuals at high risk: for example, when poor pregnancy outcome is defined as birthweight below 2500 g

Problems with dichotomizing a continuous outcome

- Information is discarded when a measurement is replaced by yes/no
- Power is reduced substantially in analyses so real differences that would show up if means were used may be missed if proportions below a cut-off are used instead
- Studies designed with a dichotomized outcome measurement need more subjects than would be needed if the original data were used

Statistical solution

- It is possible to dichotomize a continuous outcome without losing power by using a **'distributional approach'**. This works if the data follow a Normal distribution or can be transformed to Normal (see Peacock et al. 2012, Sauzet and Peacock 2014).
- This method gives both means and proportions below a given cut point that are estimated with equal precision so that the same inference is drawn from the comparison of means as for the comparison of proportions
- Both the difference in means and difference in proportions (or relative risk, odds ratio) with 95% confidence intervals are reported, i.e. a **'dual approach'**
- This is ongoing work. For the latest developments please see Odile Sauzet's webpage: http://wwwhomes.uni-bielefeld.de/osauzet/index.html.

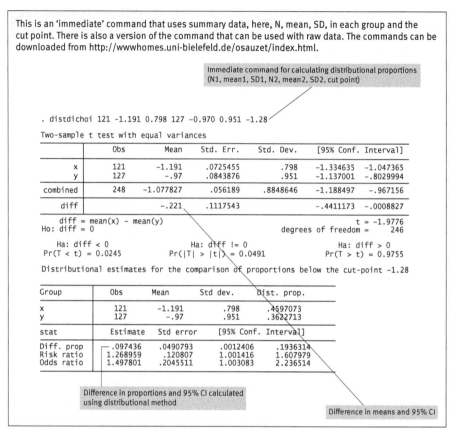

This is an 'immediate' command that uses summary data, here, N, mean, SD, in each group and the cut point. There is also a version of the command that can be used with raw data. The commands can be downloaded from http://wwwhomes.uni-bielefeld.de/osauzet/index.html.

Immediate command for calculating distributional proportions (N1, mean1, SD1, N2, mean2, SD2, cut point)

```
. distdichoi 121 -1.191 0.798 127 -0.970 0.951 -1.28
```

Two-sample t test with equal variances

	Obs	Mean	Std. Err.	Std. Dev.	[95% Conf. Interval]	
x	121	-1.191	.0725455	.798	-1.334635	-1.047365
y	127	-.97	.0843876	.951	-1.137001	-.8029994
combined	248	-1.077827	.056189	.8848646	-1.188497	-.967156
diff		-.221	.1117543		-.4411173	-.0008827

```
    diff = mean(x) - mean(y)                                      t = -1.9776
Ho: diff = 0                                 degrees of freedom =      246

    Ha: diff < 0                 Ha: diff != 0                 Ha: diff > 0
Pr(T < t) = 0.0245          Pr(|T| > |t|) = 0.0491        Pr(T > t) = 0.9755
```

Distributional estimates for the comparison of proportions below the cut-point -1.28

Group	Obs	Mean	Std dev.	Dist. prop.
x	121	-1.191	.798	.4597073
y	127	-.97	.951	.3622713

stat	Estimate	Std error	[95% Conf. Interval]	
Diff. prop	.097436	.0490793	.0012406	.1936314
Risk ratio	1.268959	.120807	1.001416	1.607979
Odds ratio	1.497801	.2045511	1.003083	2.236514

Difference in proportions and 95% CI calculated using distributional method

Difference in means and 95% CI

Figure 7.13 'Output for computing distributional proportions (Stata)'

showed a difference in mean lung function that was statistically significant but small. The clinical importance of the observed small difference was unclear. To explore this issue further, the lung function data were dichotomized according to whether the young person's lung function was below the 10th centile for normal or not (i.e. were they 'high risk'). This analysis showed that the difference between the two groups in proportions at high risk was substantial, 46% versus 36%, i.e. 10 percentage points. This is a clinically important difference since poor lung function in adolescence is associated with respiratory problems in adulthood. Hence, the data are helpfully represented by both the difference in means plus the difference in proportions at high risk. Box 7.13 shows how the results can be reported.

Note that, in the published paper, there were multiple lung function tests and only the main outcome is shown here but all tests showed a difference in the same direction. The final analyses reported in the paper were adjusted for confounding factors but gave almost identical results to the unadjusted analyses shown here. Full results can be found in Zivanovic et al. 2014.

Box 7.13 Dichotomizing continuous outcomes   *EXAMPLE*

UKOS study follow-up at age 11–14 years

Aim of study To determine whether the type of ventilation used at birth in babies born extremely prematurely affects lung function at age 11–14 years.

Study design Follow-up of a two-group randomized controlled trial.

Patient population Children who were born extremely prematurely who participated in the UKOS study and who are now aged 11–14 years.

Aim of the analysis To compare a range of different lung function measures in the two groups of children who received either conventional or oscillatory ventilation at birth.

Twenty measures of lung function were obtained but only the primary outcome, forced expiratory flow (FEF_{75}), is presented here. The remainder of results can be seen in the published paper (Zivanovic et al. 2014). FEF_{75} is analysed as a z-score to standardize for age, sex, and height.

Results: Mean z-score in the two groups

Conventional ventilation group (N = 121): Mean (SD): –1.191 (0.798)
High-frequency oscillation group (N = 127): Mean (SD): –0.970 (0.951)
Difference (adjusted for neonatal factors): 0.221 (95% CI: 0.001 to 0.441); $P = 0.049$

Interpretation and dichotomization according to high risk

A difference in mean z-score of 0.221 is small and so, although it was statistically significant, it is not clear that this is a clinically important difference. The data were therefore dichotomized to determine the percentage in each group with lung function below the 10th centile for normal (z-score < –1.28), i.e. the percentage at high risk.

Using the distributional method:

Conventional ventilation group (N = 121); percentage at high risk: 46.0%
High frequency oscillation group (N = 127); percentage at high risk: 36.2%
Difference (adjusted for neonatal factors): 9.7% (95% CI: 0.1% to 19.4%); $P = 0.049$

Comment

The difference in percentage at high risk was substantial—approx. 10 percentage points. This is clinically important. Using this **dual approach** has provided more information.

Further information on distributional method

At the time of writing this book a Stata do-file for these analyses has been written by Odile Sauzet (see her webpage, http://wwwhomes.uni-bielefeld.de/osauzet/index. html). SAS code is being written. Extensions for more complex models are underway.

For further information see Zivanovic S, Peacock JL, Alcazar- Paris M, Lo J, Lunt A, Marlow N, et al. Late outcomes of a randomized neonatal trial of high frequency oscillation. *N Engl J Med* 2014; 370:1121–1130.

> **Box 7.14   Useful references to statistical details presented
> in this chapter**   *INFORMATION*
>
> *General introduction to confidence intervals and P values* Peacock and Peacock 2011
> (chapter 8), Altman et al. 2000 (chapter 3)
>
> *Assumptions of the t test* Bland 2015 (chapter 10)
>
> *Satterthwaite's modified t test for unequal variances* Armitage et al. 2002 (chapter 4),
> Machin et al. 2007 (chapter 7)
>
> *Analysing cost data* Thompson and Barber 2000
>
> *Choosing between odds ratios and relative risks* Kirkwood and Sterne 2003 (chapter 16)

7.6 Further reading

All the methods used here are described in standard textbooks of medical statistics and we
do not list all of these. However, we think that the references given in box 7.14 are particularly useful for specific topics discussed in this chapter.

> **Box 7.15   Comparing two groups**   *CHAPTER SUMMARY*
>
> ♦ Be selective when reporting results from computer packages as they produce more
>   than is necessary to present, or is relevant
> ♦ When comparing groups, report summary statistics for each group separately
> ♦ Check assumptions of tests used
> ♦ Use a transformation if appropriate when comparing means
> ♦ Give a confidence interval for an estimate of the difference between the two groups
>   (difference in means, difference in proportions, relative risk, or odds ratio)
> ♦ Report odds ratios not relative risks for a case-control study even if both are shown
>   on the computer output
> ♦ Be careful about dichotomizing continuous outcomes and if you need to consider
>   using the distributional approach

CHAPTER 8

Analysing matched or paired data

8.1   **Introduction** *97*

8.2   **Continuous paired data: The paired *t* test** *98*

8.3   **Non-Normal data** *102*

8.4   **Matched case-control data** *104*

8.5   **Matched cohort data** *108*

8.6   **Further reading** *113*

8.1 Introduction

Matched or paired data can arise in two different ways. The first type of matching arises where two individuals are matched to each other, as in a matched case-control study. In this situation, the two individuals in the matched pair are selected to be as similar to each other as possible apart from the variables being assessed. The variable being assessed is then compared between the pair. For example, in a case-control study investigating school absence after minor injury, 422 children (the cases), who had attended a local emergency department were each matched to a control of the same age, sex, and school. School attendance was compared within the matched pairs (Barnes et al. 2001). The second type of matched data arises where two observations or measurements are made on each individual for a particular variable, e.g. lung function measured before and after exercise to investigate effects of outdoor air pollution (Hoek et al. 1993). Such studies are sometimes known as 'within-individual studies'.

It is important to use a statistical method that takes account of the matching when analysing paired data. Paired data are analysed in the same way whether they arise from a matched pair design or from a within individual design. In this chapter we will consider the unifactorial analysis of both continuous and binary paired data. We will restrict our attention to the simplest case where there is only one control per case or only two measurements per individual (box 8.1), although in practice matched studies may have more than one control matched to each case.

Box 8.1 Types of matched data	*INFORMATION*

Matched case-control studies

- Each case is matched to a control
- The differences are calculated between the matched pairs
- Thus the 'pair' of observations consists of data from two separate individuals

Within individual studies

- Two observations are made on each individual
- Differences are calculated within individuals

Notes

- Matched case-control studies can have more than one matched control per case
- Individual studies can have a series of measurements on each individual, and the number of measurements may not be the same for all individuals

8.2 Continuous paired data: The paired *t* test

The data analysed are from the Birthweight study. This analysis investigated changes in smoking habit (in smokers only) and caffeine intake during pregnancy (in all women), using serum cotinine and serum caffeine levels. These blood levels were measured in early and late pregnancy (Cook et al. 1996, Peacock et al. 1998). Paired *t* tests are used to investigate the changes. Box 8.2 summarizes the main features of the test.

The first step in the analysis was to check the distribution of the change in cotinine to ensure that it followed an approximately Normal distribution, as required by the paired *t* test. This showed that the change in cotinine was approximately Normal (figure 8.1). The results of this descriptive analysis would not usually be reported in the main body of a report, particularly if space is limited as is the case in a journal article. However, it might be shown in an appendix if the actual distribution of the variable was of interest.

8.2.1 Presenting the results of a paired *t* test

The paired *t* test tests the hypothesis that the difference in means is zero and so it is appropriate to present the mean and standard deviation at each time point along with the difference and a 95% confidence interval for the difference. Giving the individual means and standard deviations allows the reader to see the size and direction of the difference, as well as the variability at the two time points. The results of the paired *t* test using SAS is shown in figure 8.1, and box 8.3 illustrates how the results can be reported.

8.2.2 Log transformations

Figure 8.2 shows the distribution of the change in serum caffeine over pregnancy. The figure shows that these data are positively skewed, but that they are approximately

---

Box 8.2 The paired *t* test   *INFORMATION*

The *t* test is a test of significance which gives an estimate and a confidence interval as well as a *P* value

Null hypothesis Mean difference or change in the population is zero.

Most suitable for Continuous variables without too many ties (zero differences).

Assumptions Differences or changes follow a Normal distribution and standard deviations are constant across the range of differences.

Deviations from assumptions The *t* test can be used when:
- Actual data are skewed but the differences follow a Normal distribution
- Differences are skewed but the sample size is large (>100)
- Differences are positively skewed but a logarithmic transformation restores Normality
- **Note:** if data are transformed, then the individual observations must be transformed before differences are calculated

Checking the assumptions
- Does the histogram of the differences look symmetric? Note that a high peak and long tails as in figure 8.2 will not affect the *t* test unduly
- Small samples will often display an uneven distribution of differences which can be ignored if it is reasonable to assume symmetry
- A plot of the difference against the mean is a good check for uniform standard deviation (variance)

Normal after logarithmic transformation. The transformed data were therefore analysed using the paired *t* test. As for the two-sample *t* test, transforming the data changes the hypothesis being tested (box 8.4). Note that the raw data are transformed, i.e. the data are transformed *before* differences are calculated.

8.2.3 Presenting the results after log transformation

Summary statistics are always important and especially so when data are transformed. Figure 8.3 shows the summary statistics, and back-transformation is illustrated in SPSS. The key things to note are that the standard deviations and standard errors on the log scale cannot be back-transformed to the natural scale and so other measures of spread or precision have to be used. We therefore recommend presenting the individual back-transformed means and their 95% confidence intervals, which give meaningful values on the original natural scale. As we have shown previously in chapters 5 and 7, the back-transformed means are no longer arithmetic means but are the geometric means, and the back-transformed difference is the ratio of geometric means (box 8.5).

cotearly and cotlate are the cotinine levels in early and late pregnancy. This output gives the mean difference, a *P* value and 95% confidence interval for the difference. All means and error terms are given to more decimal places than required for reporting. Note that SAS gives a histogram for the differences, which allows us to check that they are approximately Normally distributed as required by the test.

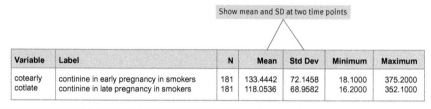

Show mean and SD at two time points

Variable	Label	N	Mean	Std Dev	Minimum	Maximum
cotearly	continine in early pregnancy in smokers	181	133.4442	72.1458	18.1000	375.2000
cotlate	continine in late pregnancy in smokers	181	118.0536	68.9582	16.2000	352.1000

Difference: cotearly – cotlate

N	Mean	Std Dev	Std Err	Minimum	Maximum
181	15.3906	52.0558	3.8693	−178.0	202.7

Mean	95% CL Mean		Std Dev	95% CL Std Dev	
15.3906	7.7556	23.0256	52.0558	47.1888	58.0509

Report difference in means and 95% confidence interval

DF	*t* Value	Pr > |t|
180	3.98	0.0001

P value

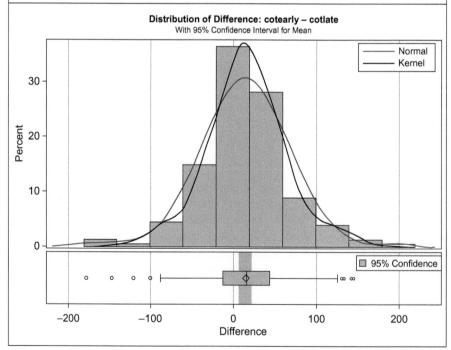

Distribution of Difference: cotearly – cotlate
With 95% Confidence Interval for Mean

Figure 8.1 Output for a paired *t* test (SAS)

Box 8.3 Presenting the results of a paired *t* test   *EXAMPLE*

Birthweight study

Aim of study To investigate effects of smoking, alcohol, and caffeine intake during pregnancy.

Study design Cohort study.

Patient population Consecutive pregnant women booking to deliver their baby at one hospital.

Aim of analysis To compare smoking intake in early and late pregnancy using serum cotinine (a metabolite of nicotine).

Table **Change in serum cotinine in 181 pregnant smokers between early (approximately 17 weeks gestation) and late (36 weeks) pregnancy**

	Mean (SD)		Difference (95% CI)	P value
	Early	**Late**	**(Early-Late)**	
Cotinine	133.4	118.0	15.4	<0.001
(ng/ml)	(72.1)	(69.0)	(7.8 to 23.0)	

Description

Methods section Changes in serum cotinine were examined using a paired *t* test.

Results section Mean cotinine level decreased by a small but statistically significant amount, 15.4 ng/ml, between early and late pregnancy.

For further information see Peacock JL, Cook DG, Carey IM, Jarvis MJ, Bryant AE, Anderson HR et al. Maternal cotinine level during pregnancy and birthweight for gestational age. *Int J Epidemiol* 1998; 27:647–656.

8.2.4 Comment on results

The distribution of the change in caffeine intake had a very sharp peak due to the women whose intake changed little over pregnancy or not at all (figure 8.2). It is likely that the lower caffeine intake in early pregnancy was a result of nausea and vomiting which was very common during the first trimester of pregnancy.

8.2.5 Extending the analysis

These data could be used to explore further the changes in smoking and caffeine across pregnancy by investigating whether changes in smoking and caffeine are explained by symptoms. For example, women often drink less coffee in early pregnancy because they suffer from morning sickness. To investigate this we would use multiple regression, which allows us to model the effect of one variable on an outcome, after allowing for the effect of another (chapter 10).

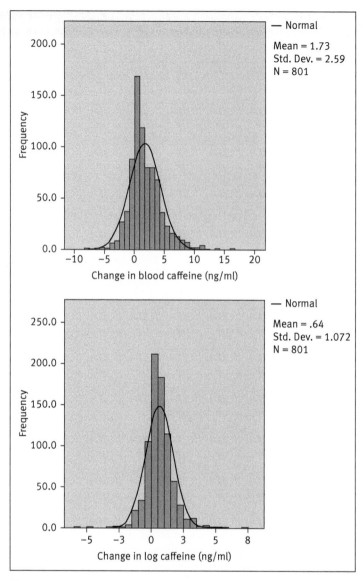

Figure 8.2 Histogram of skewed paired data (a) before and (b) after log transformation with Normal distribution curve (SPSS)

8.3 **Non-Normal data**

The example discussed in this section is from a small study of sleep in newborn babies who were laid to sleep supine and prone each for a specified length of time. Various observations were recorded in the two sleep positions, including the number of awakenings (defined according to a protocol). The difference in number of awakenings between the two positions did not follow a Normal distribution, and a logarithmic transformation did not improve matters, so the Wilcoxon matched pairs test was used. The first step was to compute summary statistics—the median and range for the number of awakenings while

> **Box 8.4 The paired *t* test on log transformed data** *INFORMATION*
>
> *Null hypothesis* The ratio of the population geometric means at the two time points equals 1.
>
> *Use for* Continuous variables with a positive skew.
>
> *Assumptions* The differences after transformation follow a Normal distribution.
>
> *Note* The standard deviations and standard errors cannot be back-transformed, but confidence intervals can.

sleeping in two different positions—and then to use the Wilcoxon matched pairs test. Box 8.6 gives some further information about the test.

8.3.1 Presenting the results of non-parametric, or rank, tests

The output using R is shown in figure 8.4. The limitation of any rank-based test compared to the *t* test is that rank tests are essentially significance tests and do not provide easily interpretable estimates. Therefore, some summary statistics need to be calculated and presented alongside the *P* value, to allow the result of the test to be interpreted. We have presented the median, the interquartile range, and the full range here (box 8.7). In other situations, either the interquartile range or the range may be sufficient.

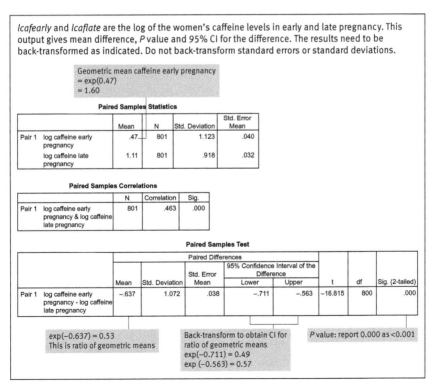

Figure 8.3 Paired *t* test with back-transformation (SPSS)

Box 8.5 Presenting the results of a paired *t* test on log transformed data   EXAMPLE

Birthweight study

Aim of study To investigate effects of smoking, alcohol, and caffeine intake during pregnancy.

Study design Cohort study.

Patient population Consecutive pregnant women booking to deliver their babies at one hospital.

Aim of analysis To compare changes in caffeine intake during pregnancy in 801 pregnant women, using serum caffeine.

Table Change in serum caffeine in 801 pregnant women between early (approximately 17 weeks gestation) and late (36 weeks) pregnancy

	Geometric mean (95% CI)		Ratio of geometric means (95% CI)	P value
	Early	Late	(early/late)	
Caffeine	1.60	3.02	0.53	<0.001
ng/ml	(1.48, 1.73)	(2.84, 3.22)	(0.49, 0.57)	

Description

Methods section The differences in serum caffeine were positively skewed and so the raw data were log-transformed. This gave differences which followed an approximately Normal distribution. The paired *t* test was used with the transformed data, and results presented as the ratio of geometric means and 95% confidence intervals.

Results section Mean serum caffeine level in early pregnancy was approximately half that in late pregnancy, and this change was highly significant.

For further information see Cook DG, Peacock JL, Feyerabend C, Carey IM, Jarvis MJ, Anderson HR et al. Relation of caffeine intake and blood caffeine concentrations during pregnancy to fetal growth: prospective population based study. *BMJ* 1996; 313:1358–1362.

8.4 Matched case-control data

The data analysed here are from a case-control study of bronchodilator treatment, and death from asthma. The cases were patients who had died from asthma, and the controls were patients admitted to hospital for asthma who survived (Anderson et al. 2005). Controls were one-to-one matched for time period, age, and area. We will analyse three drugs here, short-acting β agonists, oral steroids, and antibiotics, to illustrate the methodology, and the presentation of the data. We will only show the Stata output for one treatment, short-acting β agonists, since the principle is the same for all three (figure 8.5).

Box 8.6 Wilcoxon test for matched pairs   *INFORMATION*

Null hypothesis There is no tendency for the outcome to differ between the pairs.

Most suitable for
- Ordered categorical data, scores
- Discrete or continuous data that cannot be transformed to a symmetrical distribution

Assumptions Differences within individuals can be rated as positive or negative.

Not suitable for Situations where many differences are zero.

Limitations
- Need at least six observations (pairs) for statistical significance to be possible
- Significance test only

Note
- Analogue of paired *t* test

McNemar's test is used to test the hypothesis that the proportion exposed to the drug is the same in the cases and controls (box 8.8). The strength of association is estimated by the conditional odds ratio. Where the statistical program does not calculate this (e.g. in SPSS), it can be calculated using any program that will calculate a confidence interval for a single proportion, such as **biconf,** which is available free, or CIPROPORTION (boxes 2.9, 8.9). The details of the method are given in box 8.9 with a worked example.

8.4.1 Presentation of matched case-control data

The results are presented in box 8.10. We have shown the proportion of cases and controls that were exposed, as well as the conditional odds ratios, 95% confidence intervals, and *P* values. Note that one *P* value is very large, and was given in the Stata output as '1.0000',

---

supineawakenings and *proneawakenings* are the two variables for the number of awakenings in each position

```
> wilcox.test (sleep$supineawakeinings,sleep$proneawakenings,paired=TRUE)

Wilcoxon signed rank test with continuity correction

data: sleep$supineawakenings and sleep$proneawakenings
V = 23, p-value = 0.0003
```

Use this *P* value

Figure 8.4 Output for a Wilcoxon matched pairs test (R)

Box 8.7 Presenting the findings of the Wilcoxon test for matched pairs   *EXAMPLE*

Sleep study

Aim of study To investigate the differences in various sleep parameters according to sleeping position.

Study design Within-individual intervention study.

Patient population Twenty-four newborn babies.

Aim of analysis To compare the number of awakenings in two sleep positions, supine and prone.

Table **Comparison of number of awakenings according to sleep position in 24 babies**

Position	Median	Interquartile range	Min, Max	P value
1	36.5	30 to 40	12, 48	
2	18.5	15 to 25	10, 35	
Difference	15.5	8.5 to 21.5	−22, 36	0.0003

Description

Methods section The difference in number of awakenings in the two sleeping positions was calculated for each baby. Since the differences followed an irregular distribution, they were compared using the Wilcoxon signed rank test.

Results section The median number of awakenings was approximately twice as high for supine and prone, and this difference was highly significant.

For further information see Bhat RY, Hannam S, Pressler R, Rafferty GF, Peacock JL, Greenough A. Effect of prone and supine position on sleep, apneas, and arousal in perterm infants. *Pediatrics* 2006; 118: 101–7.

---

meaning that it is 1 when rounded to four decimal places. We have presented this as >0.999 (see box 5.1).

 We have described the association in terms of increased or reduced risk, as appropriate, and have quoted the actual odds ratio. This will approximate to the relative risk since the outcome—death from asthma—is rare, but we have referred to this as the 'odds ratio' throughout as a reminder that the odds ratio and relative risk are not exactly the same thing.

8.4.2 Comment on results and extensions

The treatments presented here are only a small subset of all those analysed, and the majority of treatments were not significantly associated with death. The published paper discussed the clinical meaning of these statistically significant findings. In addition, the case and control are the variables which denote the presence or absence of β2-agonist use in cases and controls, expressed as 'exposed' and 'unexposed' in Stata. The data are coded 1/0 for β2-agonist use yes/no.

Note that Stata gives two P values, derived from the chi-squared distribution and an exact one. We recommend using the exact one since, if the sample is small, the chi-squared P value may be too small and if the sample is large there will be little difference between the two values.

```
. mcc case control                                        Use this P value

                  | Controls                 |
Cases             |    Exposed   Unexposed   |      Total
------------------+--------------------------+-----------
       Exposed |         411          69 |        480
     Unexposed |          45           7 |         52
------------------+--------------------------+-----------
         Total |         456          76 |        532

McNemar's chi2(1) =       5.05    Prob > chi2 = 0.0246
Exact McNemar significance probability       = 0.0308
Proportion with factor
        Cases      .9022556
        Controls   .8571429        [95% Conf. Interval]
                   ---------        --------------------
        difference .0451128         .0040844    .0861411
        ratio      1.052632         1.006585    1.100785
        rel. diff. .3157895         .0880272    .5435518

        odds ratio 1.533333         1.038233     2.28449    (exact)
```

Use this odds ratio and 95% CI

Figure 8.5 Output for a matched case-control analysis (Stata)

Box 8.8 McNemar's test *INFORMATION*

Null hypothesis The population prevalence is the same under two conditions.

Use this test for two paired proportions when
- Testing the hypothesis that the underlying prevalence of an exposure is the same in cases and controls
- Testing the hypothesis that the underlying prevalence of a condition is the same at two time points
- Testing the hypothesis that the underlying prevalence of a condition is the same under two experimental situations in a cross-over study

Don't use this test when
- Testing the hypothesis that one variable is related to another
- Comparing unpaired proportions in a case-control study
- Use the ordinary chi-squared test for these situations

Box 8.9 Calculating conditional odds ratios   *HELPFUL TIPS*

Calculating conditional odds ratios

At the time of writing, SPSS gives a P value but not the conditional odds ratio and 95% CI. The following method uses the 95% confidence interval for a single proportion (section 6.2) to calculate the 95% confidence interval for the conditional odds ratio.

Suppose

- s denotes the number of pairs where the case is exposed to the risk factor and the control is not
- t denotes the numbers of pairs where the control is exposed to the risk factor and the case is not

Then

- The conditional odds ratio = s/t
- $s/(s + t)$ is the proportion of discordant pairs where case is exposed.
- $s/(s + t)$ is a proportion, and the 95% confidence interval can be calculated using:
  - **biconf** (http://www-users.york.ac.uk/~mb55/)

  or

  - **CIPROPORTION** *(https://www.crcpress.com/Confidence-Intervals-for-Proportions-and-Related-Measures-of-Effect-Size/Newcombe/p/book/9781439812785)*
- If p_L and p_U denote the lower and upper limits of the confidence interval for $s/(s + t)$ then the confidence interval for the conditional odds ratio is given by

  $p_L/(1 - p_L)$ to $p_U/(1 - p_U)$

Example using data shown in figure 8.5

Calculating the conditional odds ratio and 95% confidence interval

Using notation above, $s = 69$, and $t = 45$

Conditional odds ratio = s/t =69/45 = 1.533

Number of cases exposed among discordant pairs is 69, and the total number of discordant pairs is 114

Using biconf (http://www-users.york.ac.uk), where number of trials is 114 and number of successes is 69, gives 95% CI as 0.50937 to 0.69553

The 95% confidence interval for the odds ratio is 0.50937/(1 − 0.50937) to 0.69553/(1 − 0.69553), i.e. 1.038 to 2.284

---

authors adjusted their odds ratios for sex using conditional logistic regression. This did not affect the results substantially (see Anderson et al. 2005 for more details).

8.5 Matched cohort data

The data analysed here are again from the Birthweight study. This analysis investigated the prevalence of various symptoms reported by the women in early and late pregnancy

---

Box 8.10 Presenting the results of matched case-control analysis *EXAMPLE*

Asthma case-control study

Aim of study To investigate the effects of long-to-medium-term drug treatment for asthma.

Study design Matched case-control study.

Patient population 532 patients aged 64 or less who died from asthma, and 532 matched controls who were hospitalized for asthma. Matching was for period, age, and area.

Aim of analysis To investigate the relationship between bronchodilator treatment and death from asthma.

Table **Odds ratios (95% confidence intervals) for death associated with treatment 1–5 years before the index date, in 532 matched case-control pairs**

Drug	Case[1]	Control	Odds ratio (95% CI)	P value
Short-acting β_2 agonist	90%	86%	1.53 (1.04 to 2.28)	0.031
Oral steroids	72%	72%	1.01 (0.77 to 1.33)	>0.999
Antibiotics	86%	90%	0.66 (0.44 to 0.97)	0.032

[1] Proportion exposed to drug in case and control groups.

Description

Methods section The exposure to drug treatment in cases and controls was compared using McNemar's test. The results are presented as matched odds ratios and 95% confidence intervals.

Results section Exposure to short-acting β_2 agonists, oral steroids, and antibiotics was high in cases and controls. The prescription of short-acting β_2 agonists was associated with a significantly increased risk of asthma death, with an odds ratio of 1.53. Antibiotic use was associated with a significantly reduced risk of death with an odds ratio of 0.66. There was no evidence for any effect of oral steroids.

For further information see Anderson HR, Ayres JG, Sturdy PM, Bland JM, Butland BK, Peckitt C et al. Bronchodilator treatment and deaths from asthma: case-control study. *BMJ* 2005; 330:117–123.

---

and sought to quantify the changes in symptoms that occurred as pregnancy progressed. This was of interest because it was thought that some symptoms were common in early pregnancy and then declined in prevalence, whereas other symptoms became more common as pregnancy progressed (Meyer et al. 1994).

The first step in the analysis was to look at the frequency of each symptom at the two time points alone. Second, the symptoms were cross-tabulated at the two time points to see how many women reported the symptom at both, neither, or one time point only. McNemar's test is used to test the changes in prevalence, and the results given as ratios of proportions and *P* values. McNemar's test is testing the null hypothesis that the prevalence of symptoms does not change over pregnancy (box 8.8). Eleven symptoms were analysed

Nausea in early and late pregnancy are given by *nausea1* and *nausea2*. SAS calculates the proportions and McNemar's test. The ratio of proportions has been calculated using the BONETTPRICE spreadsheet calculator available on https://www.crcpress.com/Confidence-Intervals-for-Proportions-and-Related-Measures-of-Effect-Size/Newcombe/p/book/9781439812785;

Frequency	Table of nausea1 by nausea2			
Percent		nausea2 (nausea 36 weeks)		
Row Pct	**nausea1 (nausea booking interview)**			
Col Pct		**Exposed**	**Unexposed**	**Total**
Exposed		339	781	1120
		24.15	55.63	79.77
		30.27	69.73	
		89.92	76.05	
Unexposed		38	246	284
		2.71	17.52	20.23
		13.38	86.62	
		10.08	23.95	
Total		377	1027	1404
		26.85	73.15	100.00
Frequency Missing = 109				

Prevalence of nausea early = 1120/1404 x 100 = 80%

Prevalence of nausea late = 377/1404 x 100 = 27%

Statistics for Table of nausea1 by nausea2

McNemar's Test	
Statistic (S)	674.0525
DF	1
Asymptotic Pr > S	<.0001
Exact Pr >= S	2.436E-181

Use this *P* value
Ratio of 2 proportions above: 2.97
(95% CI from BONETTPRICE: 2.73 to 3.24)

Figure 8.6 Output for McNemar's test with ratio of paired proportions (SAS)

in the study. Results are given for all, but details of the outputs (figure 8.6, SAS) are only given for nausea since the principle is the same for all.

Note that the change in prevalence over pregnancy could be presented as the difference of proportions rather than the ratio of proportions. We chose to use the ratio since we were interested in the relative change in prevalence rather than the absolute change. In other situations the absolute difference may be a more appropriate summary of the changes (see Bland 2015 (section 13.9)). The 95% CI for the ratio of proportions is not available in all statistical programs but can be easily calculated using BONETTPRICE, one of the CIPROPORTION suite of spreadsheet calculators (https://www.crcpress.com/Confidence-Intervals-for-Proportions-and-Related-Measures-of-Effect-Size/Newcombe/p/book/9781439812785).

Box 8.11 summarizes the ways to present paired proportions.

Box 8.11 Presenting paired proportions   *HELPFUL TIPS*

Matched case-control study Conditional (matched) odds ratio and 95% CI

Matched cohort data Difference of proportions and 95% CI

or

Ratio of proportions and 95% CI

8.5.1 Presenting the results of a matched cohort study

The SAS output is shown in figure 8.6, and box 8.12 shows how these results might be presented. We recommend doing an ordinary tabulation before doing the test, to verify which way round the package has presented the results. Note that Stata can be confusing because it uses the terminology of a case-control study whenever McNemar's test is used.

The ratio of proportions is easily calculated directly from the individual proportions (0.7977/0.2685 = 2.97). The 95% confidence interval was calculated using the BONETTPRICE calculator (as discussed previously; also see figure 8.6).

Note that the matched odds ratio can be obtained by taking the ratio of the discordant cells (box 8.9; here, 781/38 = 20.5). This value, 20.5, is very different from the ratio of proportions, 2.97, and illustrates the potential pitfall in interpreting an odds ratio as if it were a relative risk when the condition being studied, here nausea in pregnancy, is common. See Davies et al. 1998 for a discussion of odds ratios and relative risks.

There was no obvious ordering to the symptoms and so we have presented them in descending order of prevalence (box 8.12).

Box 8.12 Presenting the findings for a matched cohort study   *EXAMPLE*

Birthweight study

Aim of study To investigate symptoms and health problems in pregnancy.

Study design Cohort study.

Patient population 1403 pregnant women booking for care in one hospital.

Aim of analysis To compare the prevalence of common symptoms across pregnancy.

Table **Prevalence of symptoms in early (approximately 17 weeks) and late (36 weeks) pregnancy in 1403 women**

Symptom	Prevalence in pregnancy		Ratio of prevalences %	P value
	Early %	Late %		
Nausea	80	27	3.0	<0.0001
Breast tenderness	80	26	3.1	<0.0001
Vomiting	46	17	2.7	<0.0001
Backache	45	68	0.66	<0.0001
Felt faint	40	21	1.9	<0.0001

Box 8.12 *continued*

Symptom	Prevalence in pregnancy		Ratio of prevalences %	P value
	Early %	Late %		
Constipation	40	20	2.0	<0.0001
Indigestion	36	72	0.50	<0.0001
Diarrhoea	13	16	0.79	0.0049
Haemorrhoids	11	17	0.66	<0.0001
Varicose veins	9.3	13	0.73	0.0001
Actually fainted	5.9	1.2	4.9	<0.0001

Note that the symptoms have been ordered by prevalence at the first time point.

Description

Methods section The prevalence of symptoms at two points in pregnancy was compared using McNemar's test. Results were presented as ratios of prevalence.

Results section The distribution of symptoms was markedly different for early and late pregnancy. The most common symptoms in early pregnancy were nausea and breast tenderness, which were reported by most women. The most common symptoms in late pregnancy were indigestion and backache, which were reported by more than two-thirds of women. Many symptoms, including nausea and breast tenderness, declined dramatically in prevalence over pregnancy. Conversely, indigestion, backache, and haemorrhoids all became more common as pregnancy progressed. All changes, whether they increased or decreased in prevalence, were highly statistically significant.

For further information see Meyer LvC, Peacock JL, Bland JM, Anderson HR. Symptoms and health problems in pregnancy: their association with social factors, smoking, alcohol, caffeine and attitude to pregnancy. *Paediatr Perinat Epidemiol* 1994; 8:145

Box 8.13 Further information on statistical methods   *INFORMATION*

Paired t tests Peacock 2011 (chapter 8), Altman 1991 (chapter 9), Armitage 2002 (chapter 4), Bland 2015 (chapter 10), Machin et al. 2007 (chapter 6), Kirkwood 2003 (chapter 7).

Wilcoxon signed rank test, sign test Peacock 2011 (chapter 8), Altman 1991 (chapter 9), Armitage 2002 (chapter 10), Bland 2015 (chapters 9, 12), Kirkwood 2003 (chapter 30).

McNemar's test Peacock 2011 (chapter 8), Altman 1991 (chapter 10), Armitage 2002 (chapter 4), Bland 2015 (chapter 13), Kirkwood 2003 (chapter 21).

Transformations Peacock 2011 (chapter 8), Altman 1991 (chapter 7), Armitage 2002 (chapter 10), Bland 2015 (chapter 10), Kirkwood 2003 (chapter 13).

Matched case-control data Peacock 2011 (chapter 8), Altman 1991 (chapter 10), Machin et al. 2007 (chapter 9), Kirkwood 2003 (chapter 21).

Paired odds ratio Peacock 2011 (chapter 8), Altman 2000 (chapter 7), Bland 2015 (chapter 13).

Risk difference for paired proportions Peacock 2011 (chapter 8), Altman 2000 (chapter 7), Bland 2015 (chapter 13).

8.6 **Further reading**

Box 8.13 provides references for further reading.

Box 8.14 Analysing paired data Chapter *SUMMARY*

- Analyse paired data using a method which takes the pairing into account
- Present summary statistics (e.g. means, proportions) for the two groups or two time periods, as appropriate, giving some indication of scatter or spread for ordinal data
- Present a summary statistic (e.g. difference in means, difference in proportions, odds ratio, relative risk) and 95% confidence interval for the association or change within the pairs wherever possible
- Describe the size and direction of the findings as well as the statistical significance

---

CHAPTER 9

Analysing relationships between variables

9.1 **Introduction** *114*

9.2 **Correlation** *114*

9.3 **Regression** *124*

9.4 **Further reading** *132*

9.1 Introduction

In chapter 8 we described methods for comparing two groups of individuals. In this chapter we consider the analysis of the relationship between two variables which are continuous or can be ordered, such as scores. There are two main approaches, correlation and regression, although as we describe later these are closely related to one another.

Correlation analysis can be used to investigate the strength of the relationship between two continuous variables. For example, in the Birthweight study we wanted to see how the baby's birthweight, head circumference, crown–heel length, and upper-arm circumference were related to each other. Correlation analysis gives a single index, the correlation coefficient, which summarizes how strong the relationship is (box 9.1).

Another situation arises if we want to investigate the nature of the relationship between two variables. For example, how much does peak flow rate in children increase with age? This question can be answered by regression analysis.

With regression analysis, one variable is regarded as the 'outcome', and the other as a potential 'predictor' or 'explanatory' variable. In the example of peak flow rate and age, the outcome is peak flow rate, and the explanatory variable is age because we are investigating how peak flow rate changes with age. Specifically, do older children have bigger peak flows, and if they do, how much does peak flow increase with age? Analyses of these kinds are performed using simple linear regression (box 9.1).

9.2 Correlation

Pearson's correlation coefficient is the standard method for assessing the strength of the relationship between two variables and is closely allied to linear regression. The assumptions are described in box 9.2. Other methods, such as Spearman's rho and Kendall's tau-b (section 9.2.6), are based on the ranks of the data rather than on the data values themselves, and can be used if the assumptions for Pearson's method do not hold.

Box 9.1 When to use correlation and regression INFORMATION

Correlation

• Investigates the strength of relationship between two ordinal variables
• Neither variable can be assumed to predict the other
• e.g. babies' birthweight and head circumference—how closely are they related?
• Gives a single index—the correlation coefficient

Regression

• Investigates the nature of relationship between two continuous variables
• One variable is the outcome (sometimes called the dependent variable)
• The other variable is the predictor, sometimes called the explanatory or independent variable
• Answers the question of how much the outcome changes when the predictor changes
• e.g. peak flow rate (outcome) and child's age (predictor)—by how much does mean peak flow rate increase as child's age increases?
• Gives the equation of the line—slope and intercept—which can be used for prediction, i.e. to predict the mean peak flow rate for a given age

Box 9.2 Pearson's correlation coefficient INFORMATION

Also known as Product–moment correlation coefficient.

Null hypothesis There is no linear (straight-line) relationship between the two variables in the population.

Assumptions for a significance test At least one of the two variables follows a Normal distribution.

Deviations from assumptions
• Try transforming one or both variables, as appropriate
• If transformation is not possible, use a rank method: either Spearman's rank correlation or Kendall's tau coefficient

Checking assumptions
• Plot the data to show the shape and direction of relationship
• It may be possible to see if the data are approximately Normal from the scatterplot
• Alternatively, draw histograms or Normal plots

Confidence intervals
• Both variables must be Normally distributed for the confidence interval to be valid

9.2.1 Pearson's correlation coefficient

In this example we will use data from the UKOS validation study (box 9.3). We wanted to know how strong the relationship was between two scores, both measuring the mental development of the child. The Mental Development Index (MDI), obtained from clinical assessment, was the gold standard and compared with the parent questionnaire score. These were measured on different scales. To investigate how strongly the two measures were related, the data were first plotted, and then the product–moment correlation was calculated.

Figure 9.1 shows the scatterplot. From this we can see a reasonably strong positive relationship. There is no obvious curvature and it would seem reasonable to fit a straight line to the data in the graph. We note that some R packages give the degrees of freedom alongside the correlation coefficient and P value, rather than the sample size (degrees of freedom + 2).

9.2.2 Presenting the results of a correlation analysis

Sometimes the value for a single correlation coefficient is given with a scatterplot and sometimes it is simply stated in the text (box 9.3). Summary statistics for the two variables should be given as well as the actual correlation, as shown in box 9.3.

Figure 9.2 shows the R output. Confidence intervals are not calculated by all packages but can be done by hand if needed (see Bland 2015 (chapter 11)). However, in practice confidence intervals for correlation coefficients are rarely used. Helpful tips for reporting correlations are given in box 9.4.

9.2.3 Calculating and presenting correlations between several variables

Sometimes we wish to investigate the inter-correlation between several variables. We will illustrate this using several measures of baby anthropometry from the Birthweight study.

The variables are birthweight, head circumference, upper-arm circumference, and crown–heel length. The hypotheses tested and the assumptions made are the same as in section 9.2.1 (see box 9.2).

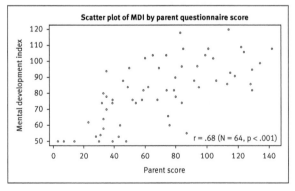

Figure 9.1 Scatterplot for two variables (R)

Box 9.3 Presenting the results for Pearson's correlation *EXAMPLE*

UKOS validation study

Aim of study To validate a new screening tool—a parent questionnaire to assess cognitive function in children. This tool, if validated, could be used in research studies to replace the existing lengthy clinical assessment.

Study design Cross-sectional screening study.

Patient population 64 parents and their children aged 2 years, who were born very prematurely.

Aim of analysis To calculate the correlation between the Mental Development Index (MDI) and the parent questionnaire score.

Description

Methods section The strength of relationship between the MDI and the parent questionnaire score was estimated by the product–moment correlation coefficient.

Results section

Table **Summary statistics**

	No.	Mean	SD	Min	Max
MDI	64	81	19	50	120
Parental questionnaire score	64	70	35	3	142

Sixty-four children were included in the study. There was a wide spread of scores, and the mean MDI was below the expected mean of 100. There was a moderately strong, positive correlation between the MDI and parental score ($r = 0.68$, $P < 0.001$).

Note An alternative presentation of correlation, a scatterplot, is given in figure 9.1. The same description could be used.

For further information see Meyer LC, Peacock JL, Bland JM, Anderson HR. Symptoms and health problems in pregnancy: their association with social factors, smoking, alcohol, caffeine and attitude to pregnancy. *Paediatr Perinat Epidemiol* 1994; 8:145–155.

Packages will produce nice compound graphs of the individual scatterplots, which can be presented if space permits (see figure 9.3 for an example produced in SAS). Figure 9.4 shows the SAS output, and box 9.5 shows how these results can be presented.

9.2.4 Comment on results

There are several possible explanations for the differences in strength of relationship between the four measures of baby size. First, they are not all measuring the same thing. All the measures are affected by how mature the baby is at birth and how well-grown he/she is compared to his/her gestational age. Birthweight and upper-arm circumference are more affected by the 'fatness' of the baby than are head circumference and crown–heel length.

Box 9.4 Presenting correlation   *HELPFUL TIPS*

- ◆ Give summary statistics for the two variables: number, mean, SD, and possibly range
- ◆ Where space permits, include a scatterplot if the relationship is unusual or a new finding
- ◆ Describe the direction and strength of the relationship as measured by the correlation coefficient itself
- ◆ Note that the *P* value only provides evidence that a true relationship exists; it does not measure the *strength* of the relationship. In large samples a small (weak) correlation may be highly significant, whereas in a small sample a strong correlation may not be significant
- ◆ Standard statistical packages do not always give a CI for product–moment correlation. A specialist package may be needed.
- ◆ When variables require transforming to meet the assumptions of correlation, the correlation coefficient **is not back-transformed**
- ◆ State which correlation coefficient has been used
- ◆ Pearson product-moment correlation coefficient may be denoted by '*r*'
- ◆ Spearman's rank correlation may be denoted by 'ρ' (rho)
- ◆ Kendall's rank correlation may be denoted by τ (tau)

---

mdi is the mental development index score and *parent* is the parental questionnaire score. Note that we calculate the summary statistics before calculating the correlation.

Present number of observations, Mean, SD, and range for each variable

```
>    with (screening,
+         describe(parent)
+         )
     vars  n     mean sd median trimmed   mad min  max  range skew kurtosis   se
1      1  64    69.53 35   68.5   68.44 43.74   3  142    139 0.23    -0.96 4.37
>    with (screening,
+         describe(mdi)
+         )
     vars  n    mean    sd median trimmed    mad min  max  range skew kurtosis   se
1      1  64   81.38 18.95     82   81.48  20.76  50  120     70 -0.1    -0.91 2.37
>
>    with(screening,
+         cor.test(parent, mdi) # pearson correlation
+         )

     Pearson's product-moment correlation

data: parent and mdi
t = 7.2976, df = 62, p-value = 6.558e-10
alternative hypothesis: true correlation is not equal to 0
95 percent confidence interval:
 0.5209932 0.7930497
sample estimates:
      cor
0.6797503
```

P value is 6.558 x 10^{-10}. Report as *P* < 0.0001.

Correlation coefficient

Figure 9.2 Output for Pearson's correlation (R)

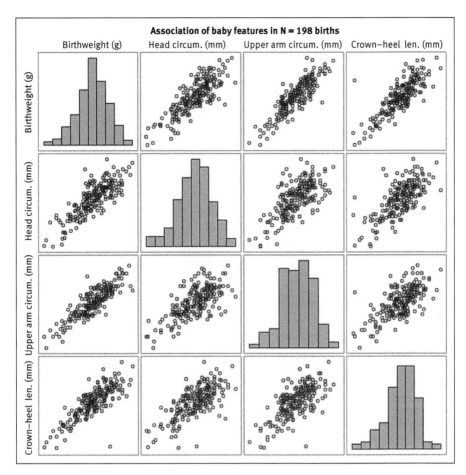

Figure 9.3 Scatterplots for several variables (SAS)

In addition, birthweight is probably measured with less error than the other measures since it is not affected by the baby moving, unlike crown–heel length. Also, the measurement of upper-arm circumference and head circumference rely on placing a tape around a particular part of the body, and so are more prone to measurement error. This illustrates that we always need to interpret any data in the light of what we know, and to try to understand why particular results might have occurred.

Note that all of the baby anthropometry correlations have very small P values and yet the actual correlations vary in size. This is because the P value is related not only to the size of the correlation, but also to the size of the sample. It is important not to judge the strength of relationship from the P value.

9.2.5 Presenting correlations when data are transformed

The calculation of correlation for transformed data is straightforward as the calculations are performed on the transformed scale and the resulting correlation coefficient is not back-transformed (box 9.6). However, the presentation of the scatterplot is affected, as we

The variables *Weight, Head, Arm, Length* represent birthweight, head circumference, upper arm circumference and crown–heel length. The option 'obs' in SAS and Stata gives the number of observations for each pair of variables. These numbers vary here as there are some missing data.

4 Variables:	Weight Head Arm Length

Simple Statistics

Variable	N	Mean	Std Dev	Sum	Minimum	Maximum	Label
Weight	198	3318	525.30744	656875	1810	4520	birthweight (g)
Head	197	351.00000	15.15767	69147	308.00000	387.00000	head circumference (mm)
Arm	197	103.81218	9.55811	20451	75.00000	127.00000	upper arm circumference (mm)
Length	198	502.30808	25.50109	99457	427.00000	567.00000	crown heel length (mm)

Pearson Correlation Coefficients
Prob > |r| under H0: Rho=0
Number of Observations

	Weight	Head	Arm	Length
Weight	1.00000	0.81236	0.87453	0.81560
birthweight (g)		<.0001	<.0001	<.0001
	198	197	197	198
Head	0.81236	1.00000	0.67815	0.69962
head circumference (mm)	<.0001		<.0001	<.0001
	197	197	196	197
Arm	0.87453	0.67815	1.00000	0.67161
upper arm circumference (mm)	<.0001	<.0001		<.0001
	197	196	197	197
Length	0.81560	0.69962	0.67161	1.00000
crown heel length (mm)	<.0001	<.0001	<.0001	
	198	197	197	198

Correlation between head circumference and upper arm circumference   *P* value

Figure 9.4 Calculating several correlations (SAS)

illustrate in figure 9.5 Hence, we will not show the calculation of correlation when variables are transformed but will show the presentation.

Figure 9.5a shows a scatterplot of tuberculosis notifications and the percentage of children having free school meals, as an indicator of poverty. These data come from an ecological study conducted in the 33 wards of Liverpool. A correlation of 0.44 ($P < 0.01$) was presented (Spence et al. 1993). Tuberculosis rate is skewed and the variability increases from left to right. Therefore, the data were log transformed and the correlation re-calculated (Bland and Peacock 2000). Figure 9.5b shows the new scatterplot where tuberculosis rate is given on a logarithmic scale, which is equivalent to plotting the transformed data. The tuberculosis rate now follows a reasonably symmetrical distribution. The transformation made little difference to the size of the

---

Box 9.5 Presenting correlations between several variables   *EXAMPLE*

Birthweight study

Aim of study To investigate factors related to fetal growth.

Study design Cohort study.

Patient population Newborn infants whose mothers were booked for delivery at one London hospital and from whom detailed baby anthropometry was obtained (n = 198).

Aim of this analysis To investigate the interrelationship between four measures of baby anthropometry.

Description

Table **Correlations between four measures of anthropometry in 198 newborn infants**

	BW	HC	UAC	CHL
Birthweight (BW)	1.00			
Head circumference (HC)	0.81	1.00		
Upper-arm circumference (UAC)	0.87	0.68	1.00	
Crown–heel length (CHL)	0.82	0.70	0.67	1.00

All correlations were statistically significant, with $P < 0.001$.

Methods section The strength of relationships between birthweight, head circumference, upper-arm circumference, and crown–heel length were estimated using Pearson's correlation coefficient.

Results section All four measures of baby anthropometry were positively correlated. The strongest linear relationships were between birthweight and the other three measures, ranging between 0.81 and 0.87. Correlations between head circumference, upper-arm length, and crown-heel length were weaker, lying between 0.67 and 0.70.

Note that there were two infants with incomplete data so that sample sizes varied between 196 and 198 (see figure 9.4 for details).

---

correlation coefficient, increasing it from 0.44 to 0.46, but that may not always be the case and so assumptions should always be checked.

9.2.6 Rank correlation

If neither of the two variables follows a Normal distribution, and transformation is not possible, then a rank correlation can be calculated. This is illustrated by repeating the calculations for the MDI and parent questionnaire data. The distribution of MDI would be expected to be Normal, but in this sample it was slightly irregular, mainly due to several children whose scores were equal to the minimum value possible (50). We will therefore calculate a rank correlation coefficient, Kendall's tau-b, for these data. Spearman's rank correlation could also be used to test the null hypothesis but is less useful as an estimate of the strength of the relationship (see box 9.7).

Box 9.6 Transformed variables and correlation *INFORMATION*

Null hypothesis There is no linear relationship between the transformed variables in the population.

Assumptions At least one of the two transformed variables follows a Normal distribution.

Notes
- Either one or both variables may be transformed, as needed
- The relationship between the untransformed variables will not be linear

---

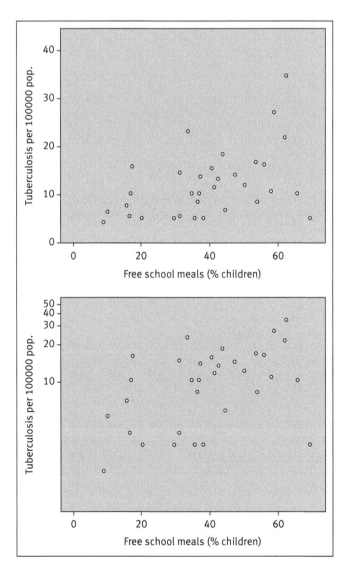

⊡ **Figure9.5** Presenting scatterplots (a) with skewed data and (b) where data are transformed (SPSS)

9.2.7 Presenting the results for rank correlation

Figure 9.6 shows the SPSS output for the calculation of Kendall's tau-b. The presentation of the rank correlation coefficient is similar to that of Pearson (box 9.3), but the median and inter-quartile range can be used as summary measures instead of the mean and standard deviation.

9.2.8 Extending the analysis

Pearson's correlation coefficient can be adjusted to take account of a third variable, by calculating the partial correlation coefficient. For example, we could calculate the partial correlation coefficient for the anthropometric data in box 9.5 after adjusting for gestational age. However, it is usually more informative to use multiple regression to investigate such relationships (see chapter 10).

Box 9.7 Rank correlation   *INFORMATION*

Spearman's rank correlation (ρ, rho)

Null hypothesis There is no tendency for one variable to increase as the other increases.

Assumptions The variables can be ranked.

Interpretation Significance test only, as rho is hard to interpret as measure of strength of relationship.

Note Calculations assume there are no ties (equal ranks). If there are many ties, the calculations may not be valid.

Kendall's rank correlation (τ, tau)

Null hypothesis There is no tendency for one variable to increase as the other increases.

Assumptions The variables can be ranked.

Interpretation Gives meaningful estimate of strength of relationship as well as being a significance test.

Note If there are ties, use Kendall's tau-b rather than Spearman's rho.

mdi is the mental development index score and *parent* is the parental questionnaire score. Note that we calculate the summary statistics before calculating the correlation.

Report *P* value as *P* < 0.001

Correlations

			Mental development index	Parent questionnaire score
Kendall's tau_b	Mental development index	Correlation Coefficient	1.000	.523
		Sig. (2-tailed)	.	.000
		N	64	64
	Parent questionnaire score	Correlation Coefficient	.523	1.000
		Sig. (2-tailed)	.000	.
		N	64	64

Correlation coefficient

Figure 9.6 Output for a rank test (SPSS)

9.3 Regression

9.3.1 Introduction

To illustrate linear regression we will use data from the Rochester study, which investigated the effects of air pollution on respiratory health. Here we use the Rochester data to estimate the relationship between age and respiratory function in 62 schoolgirls. The scatterplot is shown in figure 9.7. From this we can see that there is a positive relationship between age and peak flow rate (pefr). Regression is used to estimate how much pefr increases as age increases. Note that we put the outcome variable (pefr) on the vertical (y) axis, and the predictor variable (age) on the horizontal (x) axis. Figure 9.8 shows the Stata output. Box 9.8 summarizes the key features of linear regression.

9.3.2 Presenting the results of simple linear regression

Box 9.9 shows how to present the results. If space permits, the scatterplot may be given as well. The regression coefficient for age is given with the 95% confidence interval as a measure of precision. Note that summary statistics were presented as well as the regression results to set the findings in context. Box 9.10 gives some helpful tips on presentation.

Since there is only one regression, the findings can easily be presented in the text. If several regressions are done then the results might be better displayed in a table (see section 9.3.3).

The assumptions of Normal residuals and constant variance are not usually reported in a paper or a report. However, in some situations, it may be particularly important to justify the analysis and in such cases the results of testing assumptions should be described in the text.

9.3.3 Performing and presenting several regressions

Sometimes we wish to investigate the effects of several factors on an outcome, or investigate the effect of a predictor on several outcomes. To illustrate this we will show some analyses from the birthweight study where the purpose of the analyses was to investigate the effects on mean birthweight of the number of cigarettes smoked and the constituent content of the brand. At the time of the study, tables of the tar, nicotine, and carbon monoxide content of all UK brands were published by the UK Government Chemist.

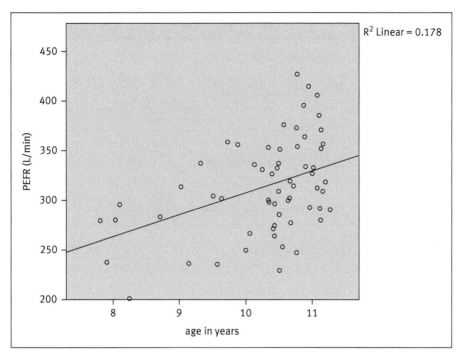

Figure 9.7 Scatterplot of two variables with linear regression line (SPSS)

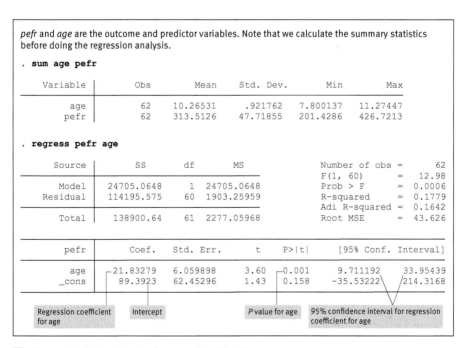

Figure 9.8 Output for simple regression (Stata)

Box 9.8　Simple linear regression　　　*INFORMATION*

Null hypothesis There is no linear relationship between the two variables in the population.

Description A predictor variable is considered to predict the outcome variable. If the outcome and predictor variables are swapped over, the regression coefficient will change but the *P* value will not.

Assumptions
◆ The distribution of the residuals is Normal
◆ The variance (standard deviation) of the outcome, *y*, is constant for different values of the predictor, *x*

Deviations from assumptions Try transforming the outcome variable.

Checking the assumptions
◆ Plot the raw data to check for linearity
◆ Draw a histogram or Normal plot of the residuals to check they follow a Normal distribution
◆ It may be possible to detect non-constant variance from scatterplot. Alternatively, plot the residuals against predictor to see if the spread of residuals varies across the range of the predictor

Notes
◆ Non-linearity, non-Normality, and non-constant variance sometimes occur together, and so a single transformation may resolve all three problems at the same time
◆ The *P* value for the regression coefficient will be the same as the *P* value for the Pearson correlation coefficient

---

We will not show any output as these are similar to those for simple linear regression (figure 9.8). We will focus on the presentation of the results and suggest ways to compare regression coefficients for different factors.

Scatterplots (omitted) had shown a negative relationship between birthweight, and the number of cigarettes smoked and the constituent content. Box 9.11 shows how the results could be presented, starting with summary statistics.

9.3.4 **Standardizing regression coefficients**

When comparing several regression coefficients, based on variables with different scales, it is useful to standardize them in some way. There are several ways of doing this. In this example, we have expressed the coefficients as the equivalent change in birthweight for a change in predictor across its interquartile range. Box 9.11 shows that the standardized coefficient for cigarettes per day is 53 g. This means that a woman whose cigarette consumption is on the 25th percentile would be expected to have a baby 53 g heavier than a woman whose consumption is on the 75th percentile. As an alternative, we could have

Box 9.9 Presenting the results for simple regression	*EXAMPLE*

Rochester study

Aim of study To investigate acute effects of high levels of outdoor air pollution on respiratory function in children.

Study design Cohort study.

Study population 62 primary-school-age girls.

Aim of analysis To determine the nature of the relationship between peak flow rate and age.

Description

Methods section The relationship between peak flow rate and age was estimated using simple linear regression.

Results section Sixty-two girls aged 7 to 11 years were included in this analysis. Peak flow rate varied from 201 to 427 l/min. There was a significant linear relationship between age and peak flow rate with regression coefficient 21.8 l/min/year (95% CI 9.7 to 34.0), $P = 0.001$.

For further information see Peacock JL, Symonds P, Jackson P, Bremner SA, Scarlett JF, Strachan DP et al. Acute effects of winter air pollution on respiratory function in schoolchildren in southern England. *Occup Environ Med* 2003; 60:82–89.

Box 9.10 Regression analysis	*HELPFUL TIPS*

- Plot the data to investigate the relationship before doing any calculations
- Check that the relationship is reasonably approximated by a straight line
- Check that the assumptions of the regression analysis hold (e.g. Normally distributed residuals). These checks would not usually be reported except perhaps in the text if required.
- Present summary statistics for the data as well as the results of the regression analysis itself
- If the purpose of the analysis is hypothesis testing then present the regression coefficients and 95% CIs
- If the purpose of the analysis is prediction, then present the equation of the line with standard errors for the coefficients
- If there are several quantitative predictor variables and/or several outcomes, consider standardizing the regression coefficients to make it easier to compare sizes of effects
- When variables require transformation to meet the assumptions of regression, *the interpretation of the regression coefficient is affected by the transformation*
- If there are several possible predictor variables, consider if there is a need to disentangle their effects and present adjusted effects (see chapter 10)

Box 9.11 Presenting the results for several predictor variables   *EXAMPLE*

Birthweight study

Aim of study To investigate factors affecting the outcome of pregnancy.

Study design Cohort study.

Study population 457 women who smoked in pregnancy and delivered their babies in one London hospital.

Aim of analysis To investigate the effects on birthweight of the number and type of cigarettes smoked in pregnancy.

Description

Methods The relationship between mean birthweight and the number of cigarettes smoked, nicotine, tar, and carbon monoxide content of the brand smoked, were tested using linear regression.

Results There was wide variability in the number of cigarettes smoked, ranging from 1 to 40 per day. Similarly, there was wide variability in constituent content (table 1). All four measures of smoke intake were negatively associated with birthweight, but number of cigarettes was not statistically significant. Of the three measures of smoke content, the standardized regression coefficient suggested that the strongest effect was for carbon monoxide content, and suggested a difference of 70 g in mean birthweight between smokers of low and high carbon monoxide yield cigarettes.

Table 1 **Summary statistics for birthweight and smoking in 457 pregnant women**

Variable	No.	Mean	SD	IQR[1]	Min	Max
Birthweight (g)	457	3204	535	3060, 3660	520	4650
Cigs/day	457	10.5	7.5	5, 15	1	40
Nicotine (mg/cig)	457	1.28	0.26	1.2, 1.4	0.3	1.5
Tar (mg/cig)	457	14.9	3.5	14, 17	4	23
CO^2 (mg/cig)	457	15.3	3.7	14, 18	3	19

[1] IQR is interquartile range
[2] CO is carbon monoxide

Table 2 **Regression coefficients of birthweight on the of number of cigarettes smoked, and the nicotine, tar, and carbon monoxide content of the brand smoked in 457 pregnant women**

Predictor variable	Regression coefficient	95% CI	P value	Standardized coefficient[1]
Cigs/day	−5.3	−11.9, 1.3	0.112	53.3
Nicotine (mg/cig)	−187.5	−377, 2.3	0.053	37.5
Tar (mg/cig)	−16.9	−30.7, −3.1	0.016	50.7
CO (mg/cig)	−17.4	−30.7, −4.2	0.010	69.8

[1] Regression coefficient standardized to an interquartile range change in predictor variable. Nicotine, tar, and CO (carbon monoxide) are all in mg/cig.

For further information see Peacock JL, Cook DG, Carey IM, Jarvis MJ, Bryant AE, Anderson HR et al. Maternal cotinine level during pregnancy and birthweight for gestational age. *Int J Epidemiol* 1998; 27:647–656.

expressed the coefficients in terms of standard deviation changes, for example, to report the change in outcome as the predictor changed by one standard deviation.

Another form of 'standardized coefficient' is reported in SPSS, where the standardized coefficient is expressed in terms of the number of standard deviations of the outcome (SD_o) as well as the number of standard deviations of the predictor (SD_p). Specifically, it is calculated as regression coefficient $\times SD_o/SD_p$. It is quite difficult to interpret compared to the methods we have described previously, except perhaps where a regression analysis has a transformed outcome that cannot be back-transformed (e.g. square root). In this situation, a standardized coefficient might be helpful.

9.3.5 Comment on the results

The analysis showed that several of the variables analysed were associated with the outcome, here, birthweight. The next logical step would be to try to disentangle these predictor variables to see if any of their effects could be explained by any of the other variables. This type of analysis requires a multifactorial approach, which will be addressed in chapter 10.

Box 9.12 Back-transforming regression coefficients *EXAMPLE*

This study aimed to explore the effect of systolic blood pressure (predictor) on cellular adhesion molecule concentration (sE-selectin). sE-selectin was positively skewed and so log-transformed before analysis.

Analysis in Stata gave the regression coefficient (95% CI) for the relationship between the log-transformed sE-selectin (ng/ml) and systolic blood pressure in mmHg:

0.00576 (0.00339 to 0.00813)

1. Back-transform using exponential (antilog): 1.005777 (1.003396 to 1.008163).

   This is the ratio of the predicted sE-selectin at any blood pressure divided by the predicted sE-selectin 1 mm Hg lower.

2. It is more useful to express this as the percentage increase per 1 mmHg change in systolic blood pressure.

   This is calculated by subtracting 1 and multiplying by 100:

   i.e. the percentage increase in sE-selectin per unit increase in systolic blood pressure is

   0.5777 (95% CI 0.3396 to 0.8163).

3. It may be useful to change the scale because a 1 mm Hg increase in systolic blood pressure is very small and, consequently, the percentage increase is near to one. It is more useful to express the increase as per 10 mmHg increase in blood pressure. This can be done by multiplying the regression coefficient by 10 *before* back-transformation;

   i.e. $\exp(0.0576) = 1.0593$, giving the percentage increase per 10 mmHg as 5.9.

Box 9.13   Presenting the results of a regression model that uses a transformation of the outcome variable   *EXAMPLE*

Wandsworth Heart and Stroke Study

Aim of study To compare cardiovascular risk factors in three ethnic groups.

Study design Cross-sectional survey with stratified random sampling to obtain equal numbers in each sex/ethnic group category.

Study population 664 men and women from three ethnic groups living in South London, who were free from cardiovascular disease and not taking any drugs likely to affect their lipid levels or blood pressure.

Aim of the analysis To examine the relationship between adhesion molecule concentrations (sE-selectin) and systolic and diastolic blood pressure in men and women.

Presentation

Methods section Plasma concentration of sE-selectin was positively skewed and therefore analyses were performed on log-transformed data. Linear regression was used to estimate the relationship between sE-selectin and blood pressure. The regression coefficients were back-transformed and the relationship expressed as percentage change in sE-selectin per 10 mmHg change in blood pressure.

Results section There was a highly significant positive relationship between systolic blood pressure and sE-selectin in women. A weaker relationship was found in men, which was only significant for diastolic blood pressure.

Table **Relationship between sE-selectin and blood pressure concentrations in men and women**

	SBP			DBP		
	Effect (%)[a]	(95% CI)	P	Effect (%)[a]	(95% CI)	P
Men (n=346)	1.4	−1.0 to 4.0	0.250	4.8	0.5 to 9.3	0.030
Women (n=318)	5.9	3.4 to 8.5	<0.001	11.4	6.5 to 16.5	<0.001

[a]Percentage increase in sE-selectin molecule concentration per 10 mmHg change in blood pressure.

For further information see Miller MA, Kerry SM, Dong Y, Strazzullo P, Cappuccio FP. Association between the Thr715Pro P-selectin gene polymorphism and soluble P-selectin levels in a multiethnic population in South London. *Thrombosis and Haemostasis* 2004; 92:1060–1065.

9.3.6 Logarithmic (log) transformations

If the assumptions of regression are not met and the data have to be transformed then the interpretation of the regression coefficients is changed. We will give an example to show how this works using data from the Wandsworth Heart and Stroke study.

The distribution of concentrations of a cellular adhesion molecule, sE-selectin, was positively skewed and so was log transformed to give a Normal distribution. An analysis was carried out to examine the relationship between adhesion molecule concentrations and

---

Box 9.14 Presentation of a regression line used for prediction   *EXAMPLE*

Rochester study

Aim of study To investigate effects of air pollution on respiratory function in children.

Study design Cohort study.

Study population 62 primary-school-age girls.

Aim of analysis To investigate the relationship between age and peak flow rate.

Presentation

Methods section The relationship between age and peak flow rate was estimated using simple linear regression.

Results section Sixty-two girls aged 7 to 11 years were included in the analysis. There was a significant linear relationship between age and peak flow rate (pefr) with regression coefficient 21.8 l/min/year (95% CI 9.7 to 34.0), $P = 0.001$.

The scatterplot and the full equation with a 95% confidence interval for the predicted values are given in figure 9.9. The expected pefr increases from 264 l/min at age 8 to 329 l/min at age 11.

For further information see Peacock JL, Symonds P, Jackson P, Bremner SA, Scarlett JF, Strachan DP et al. Acute effects of winter air pollution on respiratory function in schoolchildren in southern England. *Occup Environ Med* 2003; 60:82–89.

---

blood pressure. Box 9.12 shows how to calculate the percentage increase in adhesion molecule concentration per 10 mmHg change in blood pressure from the regression analysis. Box 9.13 shows how the analysis can be presented.

9.3.7 Prediction

In the regression examples presented in this section, we have assumed that the main purpose of the regression is to test specific hypotheses rather than to make predictions about the outcome in participants. In such studies we are primarily interested in the slope of the line and the intercept is often not reported. If, however, the purpose of the regression is to predict, then the full equation must be reported. Figure 9.9 and box 9.14 show the full equation for the relationship between pefr and age for the study described in box 9.9. A graph has been included with the confidence interval for the predicted values of pefr at different ages. The confidence intervals presented in figure 9.9 are for the fitted values. These are the expected values for mean pefr at each different age. The 95% confidence interval is narrower near the middle of the data where there are more values and so there is greater precision. The prediction interval shows the limits within which we would expect 95% of future individual observations to lie and is analogous to a Normal range for a variable. We would not recommend using these data to predict lung function in another sample, as the sample is small and there are few children aged 8–10 years.

When regression techniques are used for prediction, such as when computing centile charts, it is imperative that the regression assumptions hold and that the fit to the line is good, so that precise predictions can be made.

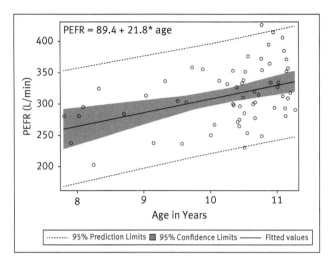

Figure 9.9 Scatterplot of two variables with linear regression line and 95% confidence intervals (SAS)

9.3.8 Extending the analysis

Where there are several possible predictor variables it can be useful to look at the effect of one variable after adjusting for the effects of the other variables. In the birthweight analysis we might wish to look at the effect of the number of cigarettes per day, after adjusting for the tar and carbon monoxide content of the brand. This can be done using multiple regression, described in chapter 10.

9.4 Further reading

The references given in box 9.15 are those that we have found particularly useful for the specific topics listed.

Box 9.15 Further information of statistical methods	*INFORMATION*
Correlation Peacock 2011 (chapter 8), Bland 2015 (chapter 11), Altman 1991 (chapter 11)	
Regression Peacock 2011, Bland 2015 (chapter 11), Altman 1991 (chapter 11)	

Box 9.16 Analysing relationships between variables   *CHAPTER SUMMARY*

- Always plot the data before doing any analysis
- Present summary statistics for the variables analysed to inform interpretation
- In the methods section, describe the method clearly, distinguishing between:
  - regression and correlation
  - product moment correlation and rank correlation
- In the results section, distinguish between:
  - regression coefficients and correlation coefficients
  - coefficient values and P value (strength of relationship is measured by the coefficient not P value)
  - positive and negative relationships
- For correlation give coefficient, P value, and number of subjects (and possibly 95% CI)
- For regression, present coefficient, 95% CI, P value, and number of subjects
- Report any transformations of the data
- Check that the assumptions of the method hold although this is not usually reported in papers and reports

---

CHAPTER 10

Multifactorial analyses

10.1   **Introduction** *134*
10.2   **One-way analysis of variance** *136*
10.3   **Multiple regression** *140*
10.4   **Logistic regression** *149*

10.1 Introduction

In this chapter we will look at how to present one-way analysis of variance, multiple regression, and logistic regression analyses. One-way analysis of variance is an extension of the two-sample t test (chapter 7) and is used to compare more than two independent groups. Multiple regression is used when there is a continuous outcome variable and several possible predictor variables and is an extension of simple linear regression (chapter 9) or analysis of variance. Note that, as with simple linear regression, the terms 'predictor variables', 'explanatory variables', and 'independent variables' are used interchangeably (box 9.1).

In this book, two-way analysis of variance has been treated as multiple regression (section 10.3.4) but we have not covered interaction terms in detail. Analysis of covariance, where we wish to investigate the effect of a categorical variable adjusting for the effect of a continuous confounder, is again covered under the heading of multiple regression (section 10.3.1).

Logistic regression is used when we have a binary outcome and several possible predictor variables and is an extension of the chi-squared method (chapter 7) and presentation using odds ratios. Box 10.1 summarizes when to use each of these methods.

10.1.1 Planning the analysis

Any complex dataset could give rise to a multitude of statistical comparisons, all with a 5% chance of spurious statistical significance. Before carrying out any multifactorial analysis it is important to identify the purpose of the analysis, decide which comparisons are of primary interest, and draw up a plan of analysis (section 3.7). This plan may have been developed when the study was designed, but sometimes research questions are identified after the protocol is written. A clear plan will help avoid being overwhelmed by output from the computer, will simplify the reporting of the results, and will help avoid spurious significant findings.

10.1.2 Preliminary presentation of the data

Before beginning to present complex analyses, the sample should be described as in section 5.7, and summary statistics should be reported for the key variables. It is usually helpful to perform and describe basic unifactorial analyses prior to doing multifactorial analyses.

> **Box 10.1 When to use one-way analysis of variance, multiple**
> **regression, and logistic regression**   *INFORMATION*
>
> **One-way analysis of variance**
>
> ♦ Used for continuous Normal outcome data
> ♦ Used to compare means from several independent groups
> ♦ Gives overall *P* value for differences between the groups, and estimates of means
>
> **Multiple regression**
>
> ♦ Used for continuous Normal outcome data
> ♦ Investigates effects of several possible predictor variables on the outcome
> ♦ Gives overall *P* value, and regression coefficient, CI, *P* value for each predictor
>   variable
>
> **Logistic regression**
>
> ♦ Used for binary (yes/no) outcome data
> ♦ Investigates effects of several possible predictor variables on the outcome
> ♦ Gives overall *P* value, and odds ratio, CI , *P* value for each predictor variable
>
> **Notes**
>
> ♦ Type of data: the predictors can be either continuous or categorical
> ♦ It is important to know the type of data and the coding as these affect the
>   interpretation of the results

The summary statistics should be appropriate for the multifactorial analysis. For example, means, differences in means, and slopes could all be described prior to multiple regression, while medians and ranges would be less relevant. Since rank methods are usually used where there are problems fulfilling the Normality assumptions, it would be illogical to follow a unifactorial analysis using rank tests with a multiple regression analysis.

When using logistic regression to adjust for confounders, it is preferable to describe the unifactorial relationships in terms of odds ratios, even though in some circumstances relative risk would be equally valid. The unifactorial and multifactorial associations are then directly comparable and show the extent to which estimates have changed after mutual adjustment.

To avoid repetition, we have not included a description of either the sample or the unifactorial analyses in the examples of presentation given in this chapter. Many examples of presenting these basic descriptive data are given throughout the earlier chapters. However, we have assumed that in any publication or report, unifactorial analyses will be described as far as space permits, so as to give the reader a better understanding of the data.

10.1.3 Missing data

As far as possible, steps should be taken to avoid missing data, but in medical and health care research some missing data are inevitable. This can cause problems both in presentation and analysis.

The data shown in table 5.1 illustrates the reporting of analyses where there are missing data. The table shown gives both unadjusted and age-adjusted relative risks for all predictor variables. Since age was available for all subjects, these two relative risks were calculated using the same set of subjects (i.e. n = 1201). However, in this study there were some missing data for the other predictor variables, e.g. ethnic origin was only available for 1096/1201 subjects, and social class was available for 1036/1201.

In order to make maximum use of the data, the analyses utilized all observations available for each predictor variable. To make this clear, the table shows the total number of observations for each of these, and gives the numbers with the various characteristics. The consequence of using all observations available for each predictor variable is that the relative risks for the different variables were calculated using slightly different sets of subjects.

If the number of missing observations is minimal, then it may be easier to produce a subset of subjects with complete data, i.e. complete case analysis. If this is done, it should be explained in the methods. The advantage is that all the analysis is carried out on the same subjects, and any differences between adjusted and unadjusted results are due to the variables adjusted for and not the subset of subjects analysed. The presentation is simpler as we only need to state the number of subjects once. In general, it is important to understand and document the reasons for missing data using baseline data, and therefore to assess the degree of bias that might arise from any missingness.

There is a growing body of complex statistical procedures for imputing missing data but this is beyond the scope of this book, which focuses on presentation. In this chapter we have chosen, therefore, to use datasets where all variables are complete, and the number of subjects is constant regardless of which variables are included in the regression models. However, note that it is important in medical research to consider missing data early in the research process, and to minimize it by good design and careful study conduct. Once data are collected it is important to consider and document the implications of any missing data in the analysis and interpretation of the results. For more information on missing data see Bland 2015 (chapter 19).

10.2 **One-way analysis of variance**

10.2.1 Introduction

One-way analysis of variance is used to compare the means of a continuous variable from more than two groups. Once it has been shown that there is a significant difference between the groups, it is often of interest to compare particular groups with each other. Care needs to be taken at this point since, if there are several groups, there will be many possible comparisons that could be made. In order to preserve the overall P value and avoid spurious significant results, the number of comparisons can be reduced by deciding in advance which subgroups are of interest and then using a method which adjusts the P value to allow for the number of comparisons made (see box 10.2).

In this section we will use data from the Birthweight study and will analyse the effects of smoking in early pregnancy on mean birthweight. Women are categorized into five groups: never smoked, quitters before pregnancy, quitters in early pregnancy, smoke 1–14 cigarettes/day, and smoke 15+ cigarettes/day. To do this analysis we first calculated summary statistics for the five groups and then did the one-way analysis of variance. Multiple

---

Box 10.2 One-way analysis of variance   *INFORMATION*

Null hypothesis The groups all come from populations with the same mean.

Assumptions
- Data are continuous
- Data follow a Normal distribution within each group
- Standard deviations in the groups are the same

Deviations from assumptions
- Try transformation
- If data are positively skewed and the SD increases with the mean, then logarithmic transformation will often correct both problems

Checking the assumptions Look at distribution of residuals (observed value minus group mean)

Multiple comparisons
- If the overall *P* value for the groups is significant, then pairs of groups may be tested
- Do not test pairs if the overall *P* value (or the chosen level of significance) is greater than 0.05
- Only test comparisons stated in the protocol, i.e. those that are of prior interest
- Use a method which preserves the overall *P* value to avoid spurious significant results in subgroups, e.g. Scheffé, Bonferroni, Newman-Keuls, Duncan
- For further reading see box 10.16

Note If there are only two groups then the *P* value from analysis of variance will be the same as the *t* test.

---

comparisons of pairs of groups were performed using Scheffé's test to investigate the effects of quitting smoking at different stages. Figure 10.1 shows the SAS output.

10.2.2 Presenting the results of one-way analysis of variance

Box 10.3 shows how to present the results of one-way analysis of variance. The mean values for the different groups are shown with 95% confidence intervals and the overall *P* value for comparing the groups. Since this *P* value was very small (<0.0001), it was reasonable to compare pairs of groups, specifically the ex-smokers. If the overall variability had not been significant, then pairwise comparisons would not be carried out.

10.2.3 Reference categories

In box 10.3, the means are presented with their 95% confidence intervals, and comparisons between categories are given in the text. An alternative presentation would be to treat one category as the 'reference' and to present the differences and their 95% confidence intervals in the table, as shown in figure 10.1b. This has been done in another example for alcohol consumption (see section 10.3.3). In some situations there is no obvious reference category and giving the means for each group is preferable, as in box 10.3. Reference categories are discussed further in section 10.3.2.

(a)

birthwt and *smokegroup* are the variables used in this analysis. Note that we assume that summary statistics giving mean, SD, range have already been calculated and reported.

Class Level Information		
Class	Levels	Values
smokegroup	5	1) never smoked 2) ex pre-pregnancy 3) ex in pregnancy 4) 1–14 cigs/day 5) 15+ cigs/day

Number of Observations Read	1513
Number of Observations Used	1512

Dependent Variable: birthwt birthweight (g)

Source	DF	Sum of Squares	Mean Square	F Value	Pr > F
Model	4	10951282.2	2737820.5	9.81	<.0001
Error	1507	420724456.9	279180.1		
Corrected Total	1511	431675739.1			

R-Square	Coeff Var	Root MSE	birthwt Mean
0.025369	15.89171	528.3750	3324.846

Source	DF	Type I SS	Mean Square	F Value	Pr > F
smokegroup	4	10951282.15	2737820.54	9.81	<.0001

Overall *P* value for smoking

Source	DF	Type III SS	Mean Square	F Value	Pr > F
smokegroup	4	10951282.15	2737820.54	9.81	<.0001

Figure 10.1 (a) Output for one-way analysis of variance (SAS)

(b)

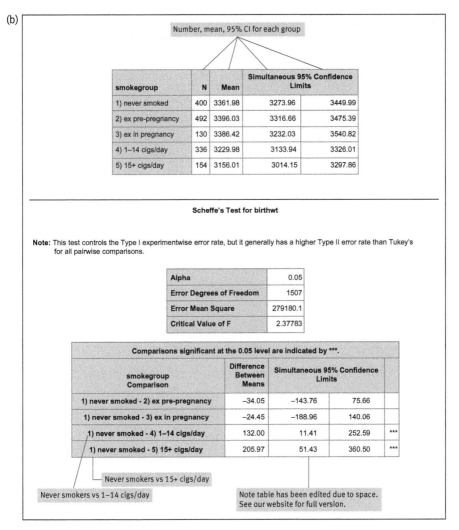

Number, mean, 95% CI for each group

smokegroup	N	Mean	Simultaneous 95% Confidence Limits	
1) never smoked	400	3361.98	3273.96	3449.99
2) ex pre-pregnancy	492	3396.03	3316.66	3475.39
3) ex in pregnancy	130	3386.42	3232.03	3540.82
4) 1–14 cigs/day	336	3229.98	3133.94	3326.01
5) 15+ cigs/day	154	3156.01	3014.15	3297.86

Scheffe's Test for birthwt

Note: This test controls the Type I experimentwise error rate, but it generally has a higher Type II error rate than Tukey's for all pairwise comparisons.

Alpha	0.05
Error Degrees of Freedom	1507
Error Mean Square	279180.1
Critical Value of F	2.37783

Comparisons significant at the 0.05 level are indicated by ***.

smokegroup Comparison	Difference Between Means	Simultaneous 95% Confidence Limits		
1) never smoked - 2) ex pre-pregnancy	−34.05	−143.76	75.66	
1) never smoked - 3) ex in pregnancy	−24.45	−188.96	140.06	
1) never smoked - 4) 1–14 cigs/day	132.00	11.41	252.59	***
1) never smoked - 5) 15+ cigs/day	205.97	51.43	360.50	***

Never smokers vs 15+ cigs/day

Never smokers vs 1–14 cigs/day

Note table has been edited due to space. See our website for full version.

📷 **Figure 10.1** (b) Output continued for one-way analysis of variance (SAS)

10.2.4 Further analyses

With smoking data, it may be reasonable to look for evidence of a dose-response effect. In these data, the never-smokers and the two ex-smoking groups were not significantly different and so these could be combined to form three groups: non-smokers, light smokers, and heavy smokers. A linear trend in these could be tested to investigate dose response. There are several ways that this could be done, but one way is to fit a simple linear regression through the groups, coding them 1, 2, and 3 and looking at the overall P value. This gives $P < 0.001$, suggesting that there is evidence for a dose-response relationship between the quantity smoked and birthweight.

10.2.5 Kruskal–Wallis analysis of variance

This is an extension of the Mann–Whitney U test to compare three or more groups and has similar properties (see box 7.5). As in section 10.2.4, an overall P value should be calculated

---

Box 10.3 Presenting the results for one-way analysis of variance   *EXAMPLE*

Birthweight study

Aim of study To investigate effects of smoking on outcome of pregnancy.

Study design Cohort study.

Study population 1512 pregnant women delivering at one London hospital.

Aim of analysis To investigate the effects of smoking on babies' birthweight and to see if those who quit smoking before or during pregnancy had higher mean birthweight than those who continued to smoke.

Description

Methods section The differences in mean birthweight in never smokers, smokers quitting before pregnancy, smokers quitting in early pregnancy, light smokers (1–14 cigs/day) and heavy smokers (15+ per day) were tested using one-way analysis of variance. Multiple comparisons were performed using Scheffé's test.

Results section

Table **Mean birthweight by smoking in early pregnancy**

Smoking group	No.	Mean birthweight (g)	95% CI	P value
Never smoker	400	3362	3274, 3450	<0.0001
Quit before pregnancy	492	3396	3317, 3475	
Quit in early pregnancy	130	3386	3232, 3541	
1–14 cigs/day	336	3230	3134, 3326	
15+ cigs/day	154	3156	3014, 3298	

Thirty-two percent of women (490/1512) reported smoking in early pregnancy. Mean birthweight varied significantly between the five smoking groups. The babies of heavy smokers weighed on average 206 g less than babies of never smokers ($P = 0.002$). Women who quit smoking in early pregnancy had a very similar mean birthweight to women who never smoked (difference = 24 g, $P > 0.99$). There was no evidence for a difference in mean birthweight in women who had quit before pregnancy compared to those who quit in early pregnancy (difference = 10 g, $P > 0.99$).

For further information see Brooke OG, Anderson HR, Bland JM, Peacock JL, Stewart CM. Effects on birth weight of smoking, alcohol, caffeine, socioeconomic factors, and psychosocial stress. BMJ 1989; 298:795–801.

---

and presented first, but medians and ranges are more suitable as summary statistics, as for the Mann–Whitney *U* test.

10.3 Multiple regression

10.3.1 Introduction

In many situations we have a continuous outcome variable with several possible predictor variables and we want to see the effects of one or more of these predictor variables adjusted for the others. In chapter 9 we showed that lung function was related to age in the Rochester study (section 9.3.1). We now will investigate gas cooking in the home to see if

| Box 10.4 Multiple regression | INFORMATION |

Null hypothesis There is no linear relationship between the outcome and the predictor variable, after adjusting for all other variables in the model.
Note that this hypothesis applies separately to each predictor variable in the model.

Use for Continuous outcome and several predictor variables.

Predictor variables These can be continuous, binary, or categorical (see the following notes).

Assumptions The distribution of the residuals is Normal. The variance of the outcome, y, is constant for different values of each predictor, x_i.

Checking the assumptions
- Plot the raw data to check for linearity
- Draw a histogram or Normal plot of the residuals to check they follow a Normal distribution
- It may be possible to detect heterogeneity of variance from a scatterplot. Alternatively, plot the residuals against each predictor to see if the spread of residuals varies across the range of the predictor.

Deviations from assumptions
- Try transforming the outcome variable. If the relationship is not linear then either a transformation may be used to model the actual relationship, or the variable may be categorized into several groups.

Cautionary note on categorical variables with more than two groups
- Care is needed to ensure these are not treated as continuous variables within a statistical package
- Section 10.3.3 discusses this

it is related to peak flow rate (pefr) after allowing for other possible confounding factors such as wheeziness, parental smoking, and age. We can do this using multiple regression analysis. Box 10.4 summarizes the main features of a multiple regression analysis.

The R output is shown in figure 10.2. In this analysis the first model (figure 10.2a) included all four predictor variables and showed that *smokers* and *wheeze* were non-significant ($P = 0.839$, $P = 0.100$, respectively). Since *smokers* had the largest P value of the two, it was removed from the model, and the regression was repeated without it (figure 10.2b). This regression showed that *wheeze* remained non-significant ($P = 0.099$) and so *wheeze* was removed and the model was fitted with just *age* and *gas* (figure 10.2c). Both of these variables remained significant and so this was the final model reported.

10.3.2 Presenting multiple regression analyses

Box 10.5 illustrates how the results can be presented. We have assumed that summary statistics would have been calculated and already presented as described in chapter 5. The results of unifactorial analyses of possible predictor variables may be presented if space permits. This would be presented in a similar way to the unifactorial analyses shown in chapters 7 and 9.

(a)

pefr, age, gas, smokers, and *wheeze* are the variables used in this analysis. The variables *gas,*
smokers, and *wheeze* are all coded 1=yes, 0=no, hence the regression coefficient is the difference
in mean pefr between those exposed and those not exposed.

```
> summary(UseAllPredictors)                    #show coefficients and p-values

Call:
lm(formula = pefr ~ age + gas + smokers + wheeze)

Residuals:
     Min       1Q   Median       3Q      Max
 -106.057 -  26.443    2.313   28.737  107.300

Coefficients:
             Estimate Std. Error t value  Pr(>|t|)
(Intercept)    75.466     60.139   1.255   0.2147
age            24.747      5.867   4.218 9.1e-05 ***
gas           -22.724     10.971  -2.071   0.0429 *
smokers         2.216     10.861   0.204   0.8391
wheeze        -24.020     14.370  -1.672   0.1002
---
signif. codes: 0 '***'  0.001 '**' 0.01 '*' 0.05 '.' 0.1 ' ' 1

Residual standard error: 41.65 on 56 degrees of freedom
  (1 observation deleted due to missingness)
Multiple R-squared: 0.2912, Adjusted R-squared: 0.2406
F-statistic: 5.752 on 4 and 56 DF, p-value: 0.0005968

> confint(UseAllPredictors, level = .95) # show confidence intervals
                 2.5%       97.5%
(Intercept) -45.00627 195.9378733
age          12.99363  36.5006567
gas         -44.70161  -0.7468291
smokers     -19.54161  23.9736903
wheeze      -52.80686   4.7671763
```

> Smoking is non-significant and has
> the largest *P* value (= 0.839). Remove
> this variable and repeat regression.

(b)

```
> summary(Use3Predictors)

Call:
lm(formula = pefr ~ age + gas + wheeze)

Residuals:
     Min       1Q   Median       3Q      Max
 - 106.984  -27.361    3.629   29.549  106.400

Coefficients:
             Estimate Std. Error t value Pr(>|t|)
(Intercept)    76.820     59.267   1.296   0.2001
age            24.706      5.814   4.249 8.03e-05 ***
gas           -22.740     10.878  -2.090   0.0410 *
wheeze        -23.527     14.046  -1.675   0.0994
---
signif. codes:  0 '***' 0.001 '**' 0.01 '*' 0.05 '.' 0.1 ' ' 1

Residual standard error: 41.3 on 57 degrees of freedom
  (1 observation deleted due to missingness)
Multiple R-squared: 0.2907, Adjusted R-squared: 0.2534
F-statistic: 7.787 on 3 and 57 DF,  p-value: 0.0001918

> confint(use3Predictors, level = .95)
                 2.5%       97.5%
(Intercept) -41.85986 195.4993410
age          13.06343  36.3495423
gas         -44.52304  -0.9573128
wheeze      -51.65391   4.5999437
```

> Wheeze is non-significant
> (*P* = 0.099) so remove this
> variable and repeat regression.

Figure 10.2 (a) Output for multiple regression (R) (b) Output continued for multiple regression (R)

(c)

```
Final model.

> summary(Use2Predictors)

Call:
lm(formula = pefr ~ age + gas)

Residuals:
     Min        1Q    Median        3Q       Max
-104.280   -30.485     6.789    29.726   112.550
```

Coefficients, *P* value for age and gas cooking

```
Coefficients:
             Estimate  Std. Error  t value  Pr(>|t|)
(Intercept)    81.417      60.118    1.354  0.180897
age            24.012       5.889    4.077  0.000141 ***
gas           -26.002      10.868   -2.393  0.019989 *
---
signif. codes: 0 '***' 0.001 '**' 0.01 '*' 0.05 '.' 0.1 ' ' 1

Residual standard error: 41.94 on 58 degrees of freedom
  (1 observation deleted due to missingness)
Multiple R-squared: 0.2558, Adjusted R-squared: 0.2301
F-statistic: 9.967 on 2 and 58 DF, p-value: 0.0001902

> confint(Use2Predictors, level = .95)
                 2.5%      97.5%
(Intercept)  -38.92189  201.755030
age           12.22353   35.800290
gas          -47.75571   -4.247918
```

95% CI for age and gas cooking

Figure 10.2 (c) Output continued for multiple regression (R)

The direction of the difference for the binary predictor variables can be deduced knowing the coding and is made clear in the table in box 10.5. In Stata, SPSS, SAS, and R the coefficient is the difference in mean outcome between the level with the highest code (here 1) and the lowest code (here 0). Box 10.6 gives tips on interpreting regression coefficients.

We have not included a table for the first analysis of all four predictor variables, but have reported the results of this in the text. It is informative to report these results to give a full picture of the analysis that was done, although, if there were many variables tested, there may not be sufficient space in a paper. We can see that, although current wheeze was not significantly related to pefr, the size of the effect was similar to that of gas cooking.

In general, it is important to describe non-significant findings as well as significant ones, because non-significance may simply be due to small numbers and there might indeed be a real effect. By presenting these data and discussing the size of effect and the possible reasons for non-significance, the researcher allows the reader to draw their own conclusions in the light of this and other evidence. As with simple linear regression, the testing of assumptions is not usually reported in the text.

10.3.3 Presenting multiple regression with categorical variables

In multiple regression we can have continuous or categorical predictor variables, or a mixture of the two. As we have already shown, categorical predictor variables with two categories, i.e. binary variables, are presented in the same way as continuous predictor variables. When the predictor variable has more than two categories, the presentation is slightly

---

Box 10.5 Presenting the results of multiple regression   *EXAMPLE*

Rochester Study

Aim of study To investigate effects of air pollution on respiratory function in children.

Study design Cross-sectional study.

Study population Sixty-one primary school age girls.

Aim of analysis To see if there was any relationship between gas cooking at home and peak flow rate after allowing for confounding variables.

Description

Methods section The relationship between gas cooking and peak flow rate (pef) was estimated using multiple regression allowing for parental smoking, current wheeze, and age. Non-significant variables were removed one by one, removing the largest *P* value first, until all remaining variables in the model were significant.

Results section

Table **Multiple regression of peak flow rate (l/min) on gas cooking and age in 61 primary school girls**

Variable	Coefficient	95% CI	P value
Gas cooking (no–yes)	26.0	4.2, 47.8	0.02
Age (years)	24.0	12.2, 35.8	<0.0001

When the four predictor variables were modelled together, there was no significant effect of parental smoking (coefficient: 2.2; [95% CI: −19.5, 24.0], $P = 0.84$) or current wheeze (−24.0; [−52.8, 4.8], $P = 0.10$). When smoking was removed from the model, the effect of wheeze was similar in size and still non-significant, and age and gas cooking remained significant. Girls who were exposed to gas cooking had a reduction in pef of 26 l/min (95% CI: [4, 48]) after adjusting for age.

Discussion points Although the effect of current wheeze was not statistically significant, the effect size was similar to that for gas cooking. It is likely that any effect of wheeze is confounded by treatment, which was not recorded.

For further information see Peacock JL, Symonds P, Jackson P, Bremner SA, Scarlett JF, Strachan DP et al. Acute effects of winter air pollution on respiratory function in schoolchildren in southern England. *Occup Environ Med* 2003; 60:82–89.

---

different. In the Birthweight study, alcohol intake was divided into five categories, and smoking was categorized as light and heavy. Figure 10.3a shows the results of a multiple regression analysis in Stata that investigated the effects of alcohol intake and heavy smoking among 456 women who smoked. This analysis arose from the observation that alcohol consumption was associated with reduced birthweight in smokers, and so this analysis included smoking and alcohol intake to try to disentangle the effects.

When the predictor variable has more than two categories, the presentation is different and also the computation/coding is slightly different. In Stata the command **xi:regress** is used instead of **regress** and in SPSS the Generalized Linear Model procedure is used, otherwise the categorical variable will be treated as continuous (box 10.7). Considerations for SAS and R are given in the same box.

Box 10.6 Multiple regression: Interpreting the coefficients   *HELPFUL TIPS*

Continuous predictor variables
- Slope or gradient of the line, i.e. the change in outcome for a unit change in predictor

Binary predictor variables
- Difference in mean outcome between the two binary outcomes. For example, if the variable is smoking, then we get the difference in mean outcome between smokers and non-smokers.
- It is important to know the coding for the variable under consideration to be able to determine the direction of the difference
- If the variable is coded 0=no, 1=yes, then in Stata, SPSS, SAS, and R the difference will be the mean outcome (yes − no)

Categorical predictor variables
- Difference in mean outcome between given category and reference category
- Stata uses different default reference categories according to the procedure used (box 10.7)
- SPSS allows lowest code or highest code to be chosen
- SAS allows any to be chosen but there are different default reference categories according to the procedure used
- R uses different default reference categories according to the package and function used

---

Box 10.8 illustrates how the results can be presented and, as before, it is assumed that summary statistics have already been reported. We have shown the regression coefficients with their 95% confidence intervals. For the categorical predictor variables, a coefficient is not calculated for each category; instead, one category is used as the reference, and all other categories are compared to it. It is important to state which is the reference category in order to be able to interpret the results.

The reference category is usually chosen by default by the statistical program unless the code is added to override this (see box 10.7). It is important to consider the choice of reference category to give a meaningful comparator and also, importantly, to ensure that the reference category does not have a very small sample size, or else all comparisons to it will be imprecisely estimated.

Note that we do not present the individual P values for the different levels of the predictor variable, but instead give just the overall P value. Individual levels of the variable may not be statistically significantly different from the reference category, possibly because of small numbers, but that is not a major concern. We are really interested in knowing if there is an overall effect of the factor, here, alcohol.

10.3.4 Multiple regression or analysis of variance?

Provided the variables are correctly specified, multiple regression and analysis of variance will do exactly the same calculations. For example, in Stata it is possible to carry out the same analysis and obtain the same results as in figure 10.3a using the **anova** command, as shown in figure 10.3b.

(a)

cigsgp is the grouping variable for smoking and has two categories: light smokers and heavy smokers. These were coded 1 and 2, respectively. *alcgroup* represents 5 categories of alcohol intake: 0, 1–19, 20–49, 50–99, and 100+g per week. These were coded 0, 1, 2, 3, and 4. *adjbw* is the outcome and represents standardized birthweight as a ratio (birthweight-for-gestational-age).

Coefficient for light smoking vs heavy smoking
(heavy smoking is the reference category)

```
. xi: regress adjbw i.cigsgp i.alcgroup
i.cigsgp            _Icigsgp_1-2        (naturally coded; _Icigsgp_1 omitted)
i.alcgroup          _Ialcgroup_0-4      (naturally coded; _Ialcgroup_0 omitted)
```

Source	SS	df	MS		
Model	.416319047	5	.083263809		
Residual	6.84185173	450	.015204115		
Total	7.25817077	455	.015952024		

Number of obs = 456
F(5,   450) =   5.48
Prob > F   = 0.0001
R-squared   = 0.0574
Adj R-squared = 0.0469
Root MSE   = .1233

adjbw	Coef.	Std. Err.	t	P>|t|	[95% Conf. Interval]
_Icigsgp_2	-.0553906	.0147751	-3.75	0.000	-.0844274 -.0263538
_Ialcgroup_1	-.0168603	.0145368	-1.16	0.247	-.0454287 .0117081
_Ialcgroup_2	-.0382412	.0155193	-2.46	0.014	-.0687405 -.0077419
_Ialcgroup_3	-.0577793	.0245754	-2.35	0.019	-.1060762 -.0094825
_Ialcgroup_4	-.0742407	.028292	-2.62	0.009	-.1298416 -.0186398
_cons	1.068829	.0150422	71.06	0.000	1.039268 1.098391

Coefficient for 1–19 g/week alcohol vs non-drinkers
(non-drinker is the reference category)

Overall *P* value for smoking

```
.
.
.
. test _Ialcgroup_1 _Ialcgroup_2 _Ialcgroup_3 _Ialcgroup_4

 ( 1)  _Ialcgroup_1 = 0
 ( 2)  _Ialcgroup_2 = 0
 ( 3)  _Ialcgroup_3 = 0
 ( 4)  _Ialcgroup_4 = 0

       F(  4,     450) =    3.53
            Prob > F =    0.0075
```

Overall *P* value for alcohol

(b)

```
. anova adjbw cigsgp alcgroup1
```

Number of obs = 456   R-squared   = 0.0574
Root MSE   = .123305 Adj R-squared = 0.0469

Source	Partial SS	df	MS	F	Prob > F
Model	.416319047	5	.083263809	5.48	0.0001
cigsgp	.213684016	1	.213684016	14.05	0.0002
alcgroup1	.214931901	4	.053732975	3.53	0.0075
Residual	6.84185173	450	.015204115		
Total	7.25817077	455	.015952024		

P values for (i) smoking and
(ii) alcohol are the same as in figure 10.3a

⌷ **Figure 10.3** (a) Output from multiple regression with categorical predictor variables using the **regress** command (Stata) (b) Output continued from multiple regression with categorical predictor variables using the **anova** command (Stata)

For further information see Peacock JL, Bland JM, Anderson HR. Effects on birthweight of alcohol and caffeine consumption in smoking women. *J Epidemiol Community Health* 1991; 45:159–163.

Box 10.7 Categorical variables with more than two groups
in multiple regression using Stata, SPSS, SAS, and R   *HELPFUL TIPS*

Stata

- Can use either **xi:regress** or **anova** commands
- **xi:regress** uses the lowest category code as the reference
- **anova** uses the highest category code as the reference
- It may be easier to use **anova** if interaction terms are required (see section 10.3.4)
- **anova** will assume variables are categorical unless specified otherwise (see figure 10.3)
- Change the reference category using '**char variablename [omit] n**' before the **regress** command, where '**n**' is the code for the category to be used as reference

SPSS

- Uses **General linear model** not **linear regression**
- Can choose reference category to be first or last
- Interactions will be fitted by default (see section 10.3.4)

SAS

- The most commonly used procedures are proc reg and proc glm
- proc reg is useful for models where the data are measured on a continuous scale and if the categorical variables are coded with 0 and 1
- proc glm provides the functionary of proc reg and allows a class statement to enable many ways to contrast levels of categorical variables
- See Walker and Shostak, *Common Statistical Methods for Clinical Research with SAS Examples*, SAS Institute 2010

R

- The lm() function provides support for simple regression modelling
- The aov() function is very useful for doing basic analyses working with categorical variables
- For many R functions you can specify reference levels for categorical (factor) variables with the relevel() function

All programs

- The reference category should not contain a small number of observations, otherwise all comparisons to it will be imprecise
- The reference category should be one that aids interpretation; e.g. it is more reasonable to choose non-drinkers than heavy drinkers as a reference category
- If unsure about how to interpret coefficients, perform regression/anova on just that predictor variable alone and compare coefficients with separately calculated group means to get correct interpretation. This is good practice as it helps to understand what the model is doing.

Box 10.8 Presentation of multiple regression with categorical predictor variables *EXAMPLE*

Birthweight study

Aim of study To investigate the effects of smoking on the outcome of pregnancy.

Study design Cohort study.

Study population Four hundred and fifty-seven women who smoked in pregnancy and delivered their babies at one London hospital.

Aim of analysis To investigate the effects of smoking and alcohol on birthweight-for-gestational-age, expressed as a ratio, i.e. the observed birthweight divided by the expected birthweight for baby of the same gestational age.

Description

Methods section The relationships between standardized birthweight ratio, smoking, and alcohol intake in pregnancy were estimated using multiple regression. The results are presented as regression coefficients and 95% confidence intervals.

Results section

Table **Effects of smoking and alcohol intake in pregnancy on birthweight-for-gestational-age in 456 women**

Variable	Coefficient	95% CI	Overall *P* value
Smoking[1]			
Heavy smoking	−0.06	−0.08, −0.03	<0.0001
Alcohol[2] (g/week)			
1–19	−0.02	−0.05, 0.01	0.008
20–49	−0.04	−0.07, −0.01	
50–99	−0.06	−0.11, −0.01	
100+	−0.07	−0.13, −0.02	

[1] Compared with light smoking (reference category)
[2] Compared with non-drinking (reference category)

There was a significant reduction in mean adjusted birthweight in heavy smokers compared with light smokers after allowing for alcohol intake. Similarly, there was a significant overall effect of alcohol on birthweight-for-gestational-age after allowing for smoking. Mean birthweight decreased steadily as alcohol intake increased.

For further information see Peacock JL, Bland JM, Anderson HR. Effects on birthweight of alcohol and caffeine consumption in smoking women. *J Epidemiol Community Health* 1991; 45:159–163.

Analysis of variance estimates the amount of the total variability in a continuous outcome, which can be explained by each explanatory variable or group of explanatory variables. These explanatory variables can be continuous or categorical. Analysis of variance tables are often displayed for regression models, as in figure 10.3a. If only one explanatory variable is used, then the *P* value from the analysis of variance and the regression analysis will be the same.

Analysis of variance treats each variable as a whole and gives an overall *P* value, while regression analysis gives a *P* value for each individual comparison of two categories.

In the birthweight example, we have assumed that the effect of smoking is the same in each category of drinking. The degree by which the effect of smoking varies with alcohol is called an 'interaction'. We have not fitted interaction terms to any of the models in this chapter.

10.3.5 Presenting unadjusted and adjusted estimates

Sometimes an analysis is performed to investigate several possible predictor variables, and this is followed by a multiple regression analysis to disentangle the effects. In this situation, it may be useful to present both the unadjusted and the adjusted effect estimates to show how much or how little the effect sizes change after other factors are allowed for. In box 10.9 we show how to present such results. These data come from the UKOS study and represent a sub-sample of infants who had a detailed portfolio of lung function assessments at age 1 year. The assessments required complex equipment which was located in one London hospital and so it was only possible to include infants who were born in or near to London. This particular analysis sought to estimate the effect of infant sex on lung function since it was suspected that boys have poorer lung function than girls, but this had not been characterized in a very young ex-preterm group.

Figure 10.4 shows the output for just one lung function measure in these analyses, FRC_{pleth}, in Stata and shows how to extract just the coefficients for infant sex to show the unadjusted and adjusted differences in mean lung function between boys and girls. By presenting the unadjusted and adjusted estimates side by side, the effect of adjustment can be easily seen. For some measures the difference between males and females increases after adjustment, while for others it decreases. Where estimates remain of similar size after adjustment, it indicates that the effect is not due to confounding by the factors allowed for. Conversely, if an estimate decreases after adjustment, then this suggests that the original effect observed was at least partly due to other factors.

Also note that in this example there are several outcomes which are measured on different scales. To facilitate comparison between these, we have presented the male/female difference as a percentage of the female mean value. This allows the reader to compare the effect of sex for the four measures, even though each is measured on a different scale.

10.4 Logistic regression

10.4.1 Introduction

Section 10.3 used multiple regression to examine the relationship between a continuous outcome and several predictor variables. Logistic regression can be used to carry out similar analyses for binary outcome variables. Box 10.10 summarizes the main features and assumptions of the method.

The strength of the relationship between the binary outcome and the predictor variable is estimated by the odds ratio, which will be adjusted for other variables included in the model. When there is only one predictor variable the odds ratio produced from the logistic regression will be the same as that calculated directly from the 2×2 table (box 7.9). For binary predictor variables it is important to be clear about the direction of the effect

UKOS sub-study of lung function

Aim of study To investigate factors affecting lung function in ex-preterm infants at age 12 months.

Study design Cohort study.

Study population Seventy-four infants born preterm and assessed at age 12 months.

Aim of analysis To estimate the difference in respiratory function between males and females.

Description

Methods section The difference in mean lung function between males and females was estimated. Multiple regression was used to adjust these differences for neonatal factors (birthweight standard deviation score, number of days ventilated, and oxygen dependency at hospital discharge) and size at assessment (length and weight). Results are presented as unadjusted and adjusted differences with 95% confidence intervals. The percentage difference was also calculated to facilitate comparison of the sex effects among the different lung function measures.

Results section

Table Mean lung function in males (N = 42) and females (N = 32) before and after adjustment for predictive neonatal factors

Outcome	Male	Female	M–F	M–F	M–F
	Mean (SD)	Mean (SD)	Difference (95% CI)	Adjusted difference (95% CI)	Equivalent percentage reduction[1]
FRC$_{pleth}$ (ml/kg)	244.2 (50.8)	213.6 (34.5)	30.6 (9.8, 51.5)	37.8 (13.7, 61.9)	17.7%
Raw (kPa/(l/s))	3.79 (1.58)	2.81 (1.01)	0.98 (0.31, 1.64)	0.36 (−0.40, 1.12)	12.8%
SGaw (1/(kPa.s))	1.28 (0.45)	1.93 (0.61)	−0.65 (−0.90, −0.40)	−0.51 (−0.80, −0.21)	26.4%
FRC$_{He}$ (mls)	212.4 (45.6)	201.3 (35.0)	11.1 (−8.3, 30.6)	19.9 (−1.8, 41.6)	9.9%

[1] Calculated as 100 × (adjusted difference)/female mean.
[2] FRC: forced residual capacity; Raw: airway resistance; SGaw: specific airway conductance; FRCHe: forced residual capacity through helium dilution.

Mean lung function was lower for males than females for all four measures, and all except FRC$_{He}$ were statistically significant. After adjusting for birth factors and current size, the differences were similar although FRC$_{He}$ and Raw were not significant. The size of difference in lung function measures between males and females varied between 10% and 26%.

Discussion points The reduction in lung function for boys is substantial and is not fully explained by differences in neonatal characteristics or in current size. The non-significance for FRC$_{He}$ and Raw is likely due to small sample size as the estimated reductions were still quite large, lying between 10 and 13%.

For further information see Thomas MR, Rafferty GF, Limb ES, Peacock JL, Calvert SA, Marlow N et al. Pulmonary function at follow- up of very preterm infants from the United Kingdom oscillation study. *Am J Respir Crit Care Med* 2004; 169:868–872.

Unadjusted estimate of sex difference (and 95% CI)			

```
. regress FRCpleth sex
```

Source	SS	df	MS			Number of obs	=	74
						F(1, 72)	=	8.62
Model	17063.9319	1	17063.9319			Prob > F	=	0.0045
Residual	142484.946	72	1978.95759			R-squared	=	0.1070
						Adj R-squared	=	0.0945
Total	159548.878	73	2185.60107			Root MSE	=	44.485

FRCpleth	Coef.	Std. Err.	t	P>|t|	[95% Conf. Interval]	
sex	-30.65179	10.43841	-2.94	0.004	-51.46038	-9.84319
_cons	274.8661	15.82133	17.37	0.000	243.3268	306.4053

```
. regress FRCpleth sex sds 1daysvent o2depdis length weight
```

Source	SS	df	MS			Number of obs	=	74
						F(6, 67)	=	2.67
Model	30791.548	6	5131.92467			Prob > F	=	0.0220
Residual	128757.33	67	1921.7512			R-squared	=	0.1930
						Adj R-squared	=	0.1207
Total	159548.878	73	2185.60107			Root MSE	=	43.838

FRCpleth	Coef.	Std. Err.	t	P>|t|	[95% Conf. Interval]	
sex	-37.79622	12.0918	-3.13	0.003	-61.93156	-13.66089
sds	.865532	5.792757	0.15	0.882	-10.69686	12.42792
1daysvent	-.3882754	4.365722	-0.09	0.929	-9.102292	8.325742
o2depdis	-9.024777	14.16577	-0.64	0.526	-37.29977	19.25022
length	4.678955	2.586894	1.81	0.075	-.4845077	9.842418
weight	.61826	6.229929	0.10	0.921	-11.81673	13.05325
_cons	-49.15526	153.0794	-0.32	0.749	-354.703	256.3925

Adjusted estimate of sex difference (and 95% CI)			

Figure 10.4 Output for multiple regression (Stata)

For further information see Greenough A, Limb E, Marston L, Marlow N, Calvert S, Peacock J. Risk factors for respiratory morbidity in infancy after very premature birth. *Arch Dis Child Fetal Neonatal Ed* 2005; 90:F320–F323

(box 10.11). For continuous predictors the odds ratio obtained is the odds of outcome for a unit change in predictor. More details are given in box 10.11.

To illustrate the presentation of logistic regression, we will use data from the UKOS study. The data come from a clinical follow-up at age 1 year, and this analysis looks at the relationship between neonatal factors and the prescribing of chest medicines at 1 year of age. Eight neonatal variables were initially examined in unifactorial analyses to determine whether they were associated with chest medicines. The four variables that were significant at the 5% level (sex, multiple birth, oxygen dependency at 36 weeks postmenstrual age, oxygen dependency at hospital discharge) were then put in a logistic regression model to try to disentangle the effects. Figure 10.5 shows the SPSS output. Some packages, e.g. SAS, show the c-statistic, or area under the receiver operating curve, 0.65 in this example. This indicates that the predictive power of this set of variables is only moderately strong.

> **Box 10.10 Logistic regression**   *INFORMATION*
>
> *Null hypothesis* There is no relationship between the outcome and the predictor
> variable, after adjusting for all other variables in the model.
> Note this hypothesis applies separately to each predictor variable in the model.
>
> *Use for* Binary outcome and several predictor variables.
>
> *Predictor variables* These can be continuous, binary, or categorical.
>
> *Assumptions*
> - For continuous predictors only, the relationship is linear on the logit scale
> - Large-sample method. Rule-of-thumb is that the analysis requires at least 10
>   positives and 10 negatives per predictor variable (Peduzzi et al. 1996).
>
> *Deviations from assumptions*
> - If the relationship is not linear then either a transformation of the predictor variable
>   may be used to model the actual relationship or the predictor variable may be
>   categorized into several groups
> - If sample is too small, use an exact method (available in Stata, SAS, and R) but be
>   aware that this will be computationally intensive

10.4.2 Presenting the results of logistic regression

Box 10.12 shows how to present the results. The overall number and percentage of babies
prescribed chest medicines is reported to give an estimate of the overall risk and shows that
the number of events is sufficiently large for a robust logistic regression analysis. Summary
statistics for the study are not given here to save space, but would be included before the
logistic regression results in a full paper or report. We have given the odds ratio, 95% confidence interval, and *P* value in a table. The direction of effect for sex of infant (male/female)
has been explicitly stated to avoid any uncertainty. For the yes/no variables, it is assumed
that the odds ratio is for yes vs no. In the description we have indicated the size of effect
and stated that the odds ratios are adjusted for the other variables in the model to distinguish these results from ordinary variable-by-variable results (unadjusted results). We will
give an example of presenting unadjusted and adjusted results together in section 10.4.4.

10.4.3 Presenting logistic regression with categorical predictor variables

The key features of the presentation of categorical variables in logistic regression are similar to those for multiple regression (section 10.3.3). Overall *P* values should be presented
and care needs to be taken to obtain and describe the appropriate reference category
(box 10.13) Packages will assume that predictor variables are continuous unless otherwise
specified as in figure 10.6, where to generate this analysis in SPSS the 'categorical' box needs
to be checked.

To illustrate, we investigate the relationship between nausea and smoking and social
class from the Birthweight study. This analysis is related to that shown in section 8.5. In
the unifactorial analysis we used relative risk to describe the relationships. Here we will

---

Box 10.11 Logistic regression: Interpretation of coefficients   *HELPFUL TIPS*

Log odds ratios
- The coefficients from logistic regression are log odds ratios
- These must be back-transformed (take exponential) to give odds ratios
- Packages will do this for you, or do by hand with a computer or calculator
- Below we assume coefficients have been back-transformed

Binary predictor variables
- These give the odds ratio for the outcome in the two levels of the predictor variable. For example, if the outcome is death, and the predictor variable is smoking, then we get the ratio of odds of dying in smokers vs non-smokers.
- Note it is important to know the coding for the variable under consideration to be able to determine the direction of the difference
- If all variables are coded 0=no, 1=yes, then the odds ratio will be the odds of the outcome in the 'yes' group divided by the odds of the outcome in the 'no' group (yes/no)

Categorical predictor variables
- These give the odds ratio for the outcome in a given category divided by the odds of the outcome in the reference category
- Check how the package decides which is the reference category (see box 10.7 for discussion of reference values in multiple regression)

Continuous predictor variables
- The odds ratio is the change in the odds of the outcome for a unit change in the predictor
- For example, if the outcome was death, and the predictor was the number of packs of cigarettes smoked per day, then the odds ratio would be for 2 packs/day vs 1 pack/day. This is the same as 3 packs/day vs 2 packs/day, etc.
- If the odds ratio is 1.5, then 4 packs/day vs 1 pack/day would be obtained by taking $1.5 \times 1.5 \times 1.5 = 1.5^3 = 3.4$

---

use odds ratios because the analysis is more straightforward than one which attempts to adjust the relative risks, especially as the outcome is common (see box 7.9). Smoking habit is divided into three categories: non-smoker, light smoker, and heavy smoker. The SPSS output is shown in figure 10.6, and the presentation is in box 10.14.

Odds ratios, 95% confidence intervals, and *P* values are reported. The overall *P* value for smoking is given alongside the reference category, and the 95% confidence intervals are given for each comparison. The direction of the effects is clear because we have indicated the reference category against which all other categories are compared. Note that in this example the reference category is indicated by the odds ratio of 1.0. If space is limited, the reference category can be indicated in a footnote, as in box 10.8.

We have described the direction of the effects and stated that these are *adjusted*. It is important to say this if there is any possibility of ambiguity, for example, when unadjusted and adjusted effects are described together. If it is obvious that the odds ratios are adjusted *chest* (outcome), *sex, multiple,* and *o2dep36w, and o2depdis* (predictors) are the variables. All variables were coded 0=no, 1=yes, except sex, where 0=female, 1=male.

Omnibus Tests of Model Coefficients

		Chi-square	df	Sig.
Step 1	Step	31.796	4	.000
	Block	31.796	4	.000
	Model	31.796	4	.000

Model Summary

Step	−2 Log likelihood	Cox & Snell R Square	Nagelkerke R Square
1	534.105[a]	.072	.098

a. Estimation terminated at iteration number 4 because parameter estimates changed by less than .001.

o2depdis is not significant so repeat analysis without it

Variables in the Equation

		B	S.E.	Wald	df	Sig.	Exp(B)	95% C.I. for Exp(B) Lower	Upper
Step 1[a]	sex	.419	.210	3.980	1	.046	1.521	1.007	2.296
	multiple	−.788	.267	8.687	1	.003	.455	.269	.768
	o2dep36w	.516	.236	4.770	1	.029	1.676	1.054	2.663
	o2depdis	.529	.276	3.679	1	.055	1.697	.989	2.914
	Constant	−.956	.198	23.240	1	.000	.385		

a. Variable(s) entered on step 1: sex, multiple, o2dep36w, o2depdis.

Variables in the Equation

		B	S.E.	Wald	df	Sig.	Exp(B)	95% C.I. for Exp(B) Lower	Upper
Step 1[a]	sex	.416	.207	4.019	1	.045	1.516	1.009	2.276
	multiple	−.810	.266	9.275	1	.002	.446	.264	.749
	o2dep36w	.727	.213	11.637	1	.001	2.069	1.363	3.143
	Constant	−.958	.197	23.673	1	.000	.383		

a. Variable(s) entered on step 1: sex, multiple, o2dep36w.

Odds ratio for sex, *P* value, and 95% CI. Odds ratio for multiple and *o2dep36w* are in second and third rows

Figure 10.5 Output for logistic regression (SPSS)

For further information see Greenough A, Limb E, Marston L, Marlow N, Calvert S, Peacock J. Risk factors for respiratory morbidity in infancy after very premature birth. *Arch Dis Child Fetal Neonatal Ed* 2005; 90:F320–F323

then a simple statement that all effect estimates are adjusted for all other variables in the model is sufficient.

We have described the results in terms which do not imply causality since this is an observational study where the outcome and exposures are occurring concurrently. It would, of course, be wrong to state, or imply, that this analysis shows that smoking and manual social class protect against nausea in pregnancy. The relationship *may* be causal, but it is more likely that smoking and manual social class are markers for women who do not tend to get nausea for other reasons. Another possibility is that that women who have nausea stop smoking. This study and this analysis cannot distinguish between these possibilities and we have to be careful how we describe and present the results so as not to mislead the reader.

Box 10.12 Presenting the results for logistic regression   *EXAMPLE*

UKOS study

Aim of study To assess the respiratory health of infants at age 1 year following very premature birth.

Study design Follow-up of surviving babies from a randomized controlled trial.

Study population Four hundred and twenty-nine surviving infants.

Aim of analysis To investigate the effect of neonatal factors on the use of chest medicines at age 1 year.

Description

Methods section The combined effect of four neonatal variables that were significantly related to the use of chest medicines at age 1 year (sex, single/multiple birth, oxygen dependency at 36 weeks postmenstrual age, oxygen dependency at hospital discharge) were investigated using logistic regression. Results are presented as odds ratios and 95% confidence intervals.

Results section

Table **Adjusted[1] odds ratios for effects of neonatal variables on use of chest medicines at age 1 year in 316 infants**

Variable	Odds ratio	95% CI	*P* value
Sex (male/female)	1.52	1.01, 2.28	0.045
Multiple birth	0.45	0.26, 0.75	0.002
O_2 dependency at 36w PMA[2]	2.07	1.36, 3.14	0.001

[1] Each odds ratio is adjusted for all other variables in the table
[2] PMA: postmenstrual age

One hundred and sixty-five babies (38%) were prescribed chest medicines at age 1 year. The proportion prescribed was higher in males than females (45% vs 32%), lower in multiple births than singletons (25% vs 42%), and higher in those who were oxygen dependent at 36 weeks PMA (46% vs 28%) and in those who were oxygen dependent at hospital discharge (55% vs 34%).

When the four significant neonatal variables were analysed together, oxygen dependency at hospital discharge became non-significant (OR 1.70, 95% CI 0.99, 2.91) but the other three factors remained significant. After adjustment, male sex was associated with a 50% increase in odds of use of chest medicines, while multiple birth was associated with a halving of the odds. Oxygen dependency at 36 weeks PMA was associated with more than double the odds of prescription of chest medicines.

For further information see Greenough A, Limb E, Marston L, Marlow N, Calvert S, Peacock J. Risk factors for respiratory morbidity in infancy after very premature birth. *Arch Dis Child Fetal Neonatal Ed* 2005; 90:F320–F323.

Box 10.13 Categorical variables in logistic regression   *INFORMATION*

Stata

- Uses **xi:logistic** and **i.variable** to identify the categorical variables
- It uses the lowest category code as the reference
- You need to use the likelihood ratio test to get the overall *P* value for the three-category factor.For example, the following code will give the overall *P* value for the three-category variable 'smoker1' . Note that, since social class has just two categories, the *P* value is automatically given (see model in figure 10.6):
  - **xi:logistic nausea1 i.smoker1 i.socialclass**
  - **estimates store a**
  - **xi:logistic nausea i.socialclass**
  - **estimates store b**
  - **lrtest a b**

SPSS

- Uses **categorical** option to identify categorical variables
- Can choose reference category to be first or last
- Gives overall *P* value by default

SAS

- Must use **class** option to identify categorical variables
- Can choose reference category
- Gives overall *P* value by default

R

- Uses a **factor()** function to identify categorical variables
- Uses lowest category code as the reference
- Needs to do likelihood ratio test to get overall *P* value; see http://ww2.coastal.edu/kingw/statistics/R-tutorials/logistic.html for help

All programs

- Binary variables need not be identified as categorical
- The reference category should not contain a small number of observations
- The reference category should be one that makes sense; e.g. it is more reasonable to choose non-smokers than heavy smokers as a reference category

---

10.4.4 Presenting unadjusted and adjusted odds ratios

Sometimes, it may be informative to present both the unadjusted estimates and the adjusted estimates obtained from a multifactorial analysis. This can be useful to show how estimates change after adjustment. Box 10.15 shows an extract of a table from the UKOS study, which was reporting the predictors of respiratory symptoms in infants. Several variables were

The variables used in this analysis are *nausea1*, *smoker1*, and *socialclass*. *nausea1* is coded 0, 1 (no/yes), and *smoker1* is coded 0, 1, 2 (non-smoker, light smoker, heavy smoker). *socialclass* is coded 0, 1 (non-manual/manual).

Case Processing Summary

Unweighted Cases[a]		N	Percent
Selected Cases	Included in Analysis	1469	97.1
	Missing Cases	44	2.9
	Total	1513	100.0
Unselected Cases		0	.0
Total		1513	100.0

a. If weight is in effect, see classification table for the total number of cases.

Omnibus Tests of Model Coefficients

		Chi-square	df	Sig.
Step 1	Step	24.890	3	.000
	Block	24.890	3	.000
	Model	24.890	3	.000

Model Summary

Step	−2 Log likelihood	Cox & Snell R Square	Nagelkerke R Square
1	1467.744[a]	.017	.026

a. Estimation terminated at iteration number 4 because parameter estimates changed by less than .001.

Odds ratio for light smokers vs non-smokers (reference category)

Variables in the Equation

		B	S.E.	Wald	df	Sig.	Exp(B)	95% C.I. for Exp(B)	
								Lower	Upper
Step 1[a]	smoker1			17.399	2	.000			
	smoker1(1)	−.523	.153	11.764	1	.001	.593	.439	.799
	smoker1(2)	−.633	.200	9.991	1	.002	.531	.359	.786
	socialclass(1)	−.319	.158	4.076	1	.043	.727	.534	.991
	Constant	1.077	.085	159.507	1	.000	2.934		

a. Variable(s) entered on step 1: smoker1, socialclass.

P value for overall effect of smoking

P value for social class and odds ratio (95% CI) for manual vs non-manual (reference category)

Figure 10.6 Output for logistic regression with categorical predictor variables (SPSS)

For further information see Peacock JL, Cook DG, Carey IM, Jarvis MJ, Bryant AE, Anderson HR et al. Maternal cotinine level during pregnancy and birthweight for gestational age. *Int J Epidemiol* 1998; 27:647–656

associated with adverse symptoms when examined in unifactorial analyses, and it was interesting to see that the strengths of the relationships did not change much after mutual adjustment. As commented in the box, this suggests that the predictors were acting independently of each other. If alternatively, for example, one estimate had been much smaller after adjustment, this would have suggested that part of its observed effect when examined alone was in fact due to the other variables in the model.

Box 10.14 Presenting logistic regression with categorical predictor variables   *EXAMPLE*

Birthweight study

Aim of study To investigate symptoms and health problems in pregnancy.

Study design Cohort study.

Study population One thousand four hundred and sixty-nine pregnant women booked to deliver their babies at one London hospital.

Aim of analysis To investigate the relationship between nausea in pregnancy and mother's smoking habit and her socioeconomic status.

Description

Methods section The effects of smoking and social class on nausea in early pregnancy were investigated using logistic regression. Results are presented as odds ratios and 95% confidence intervals.

Results section

Table **Adjusted odds ratios for the effects of smoking and social class on nausea in early pregnancy in 1469 women**

Variable	Odds ratio[1]	95% CI	P value
Smoking			
Non-smoker[2]	1.0		<0.001
Light smoker	0.59	0.44, 0.80	
Heavy smoker	0.53	0.36, 0.79	
Social class			
Non-manual[2]	1.0		0.04
Manual	0.73	0.53, 0.99	

[1] Adjusted for the other variables in the table
[2] Reference category

Overall, the majority of women (1167/1469, 79%) reported nausea during the first trimester of pregnancy. However, nausea was significantly less common in smokers than non-smokers (72% vs 83%) and was less common in women in manual occupations than non-manual (73% vs 81%).

After mutual adjustment, both smoking and social class remained significantly associated with nausea in pregnancy. After adjustment for social class, both light and heavy smoking were associated with reduced odds of nausea compared with not smoking. Conversely, after adjustment for smoking, women in manual occupations had reduced odds of nausea than those in non-manual occupations.

When reporting unadjusted and adjusted estimates together, it may not be necessary to give confidence intervals for the unadjusted estimates if space is limited, but confidence intervals should be given for the adjusted estimates. Another example of presenting unadjusted and adjusted estimates was given in table 5.1.

Box 10.16 gives further information on the statistical methods used in this chapter.

Box 10.15 Presenting unadjusted and adjusted logistic regression   *EXAMPLE*

Description

Results section

Table **Factors related to cough and wheeze reported at both 6 and 12 months of age estimated in logistic regression analysis**

Outcome	Predictor variables	Unadjusted OR	Adjusted OR	(95% CI)
Cough	Sex: boy	1.80	1.83	1.11, 3.02
	Oxygen dependent at discharge	2.01	1.76	1.00, 3.11
	Live in rented accommodation	1.96	1.67	1.02, 2.73
	Older siblings aged <5 years	1.70	2.25	1.34, 3.80
Wheeze	Multiple birth	0.36	0.37	0.18, 0.77
	Oxygen dependent at 36 wk PMA	2.43	2.74	1.55, 4.83
	Pet ownership	0.42	0.43	0.21, 0.87
	Older siblings aged <5 years	1.54	1.98	1.13, 3.49

Four factors were significantly associated with cough. Male sex, oxygen dependency at hospital discharge, living in rented accommodation, and having older siblings under the age of 5 years were associated with 1.7- to 2-fold increases in odds of cough. For wheeze, predictive factors were oxygen dependency at 36 weeks postmenstrual age and older siblings, showing 1.5- to over 2-fold increases in odds. Multiple birth and pet ownership showed inverse (protective) associations with wheeze. Unadjusted and adjusted odds ratios were very similar.

Discussion points The similarity of the unadjusted and adjusted odds ratios suggests that these factors are acting independently of each other.

For further information see Greenough A, Limb E, Marston L, Marlow N, Calvert S, Peacock J. Risk factors for respiratory morbidity in infancy after very premature birth. *Arch Dis Child Fetal Neonatal Ed* 2005; 90:F320-F323.

Box 10.16 Further information on statistical methods   *INFORMATION*

One-way analysis of variance Peacock 2011 (chapter 8), Bland 2015 (chapter 10), Altman 1991 (chapter 9)

Multiple comparisons Bland 2015 (chapter 9), Altman 1991 (chapter 9), Peacock 2011 (chapter 8)

Multiple regression Peacock 2011 (chapter 12), Bland 2015 (chapter 15), Altman 1991 (chapter 12)

Logistic regression Peacock 2011 (chapter 12), Bland 2015 (chapter 15), Altman 1991 (chapter 12)

Missing data Bland 2015 (chapter 19), Peacock 2011 (chapter 12)

Box 10.17 Multifactorial analyses   *CHAPTER SUMMARY*

- Plan the analysis beforehand and present what you find even if the results are not statistically significant
- Present summary statistics for the variables included as appropriate to the analysis conducted
- Make sure categorical and continuous variables are specified correctly in the statistical program used
- Make and report on appropriate adjustment for any multiple comparisons
- Present adjusted slopes, adjusted difference in means, or adjusted odds ratios as appropriate, with their 95% CIs
- Report all of the variables included in the models fitted
- Unless it is obvious, specify how the variables have been modelled; e.g. with age, it could be modelled as a continuous variable with a linear relationship, as a quadratic relationship or treated as categorical (what categories), etc.
- State clearly any reference categories and the direction of all effects/differences
- Give the overall P value for any categorical variable with more than two groups
- Report any transformations of the data
- Check that the assumptions of the methods used hold, although this is not usually reported in papers and reports

---

CHAPTER 11

Survival analysis

11.1   **Introduction** *161*

11.2   **Kaplan–Meier estimates of survival rates** *165*

11.3   **The logrank test** *165*

11.4   **Cox regression** *166*

11.5   **Further reading** *172*

11.1 Introduction

In the Peripheral Vascular Disease study (box 7.2), subjects have been classified into those who died and those who survived. Another way of looking at these data is to see how long patients survived. Although commonly referred to as 'survival' analysis, these methods are more generally described as 'time-to-event' analyses. The methods take account of the different lengths of time subjects have been followed up without experiencing an event (see box 11.1).

In studies where all subjects have experienced an event and no subjects are lost to follow-up, the time to event may be analysed using methods described earlier in the book (chapter 7). Since time to event is often highly skewed, a transformation followed by a *t* test or a rank test such as a Mann–Whitney *U* test may be appropriate. For example, in a trial of a drug to resolve symptoms for sore throat in healthy individuals, all participants will experience a resolution of their symptoms (the event), and so the length of time to resolution in different groups can be directly compared.

In this chapter we will describe Kaplan–Meier methods for displaying the survival curve and estimating survival rates, the logrank test, and Cox regression. There are other methods for estimating survival rates, such as Weibull regression, but Cox regression is the most commonly seen. For a more detailed discussion of various methods see Machin et al. 2007 and Machin et al. 2006.

An alternative to the Kaplan–Meier method is the life table method, which assumes that events are known to take place within a time period rather than taking place at a certain time. If life table methods are used with a small interval then they will give the same results as Kaplan–Meier methods. There are a few situations where the life table procedures may be useful and these are given in box 11.2.

11.1.1 Description of the study sample

The report of the results of survival analysis should start with a description of the sample. This should include the total sample size, the total number of events, and the average (mean or median) follow-up time, as well as some measure of variability in the follow-up

> **Box 11.1 Uses of survival methods**   *INFORMATION*
>
> *Used for time to any event* Many different events can be studied using 'survival methods' but time to death is the most commonly analysed. Others include time to disease recurrence, time to first cardiovascular event (fatal or non-fatal), time to recovery/healing, and time to conception.
>
> *Number of events per person* Standard statistical procedures assume by default that there is a maximum of one event per person. Hence, if multiple events per individual are possible, such as with non-fatal cardiovascular events, then the time to the first event might be chosen for analysis.
>
> Multiple events per person can be analysed but this is not straightforward, see Collett (chapter 13). We recommend seeking statistical help for the analysis of multiple events.
>
> *Censored observations* Survival methods make allowance for incomplete follow-up of subjects. All subjects who have not experienced the event are 'censored' at the last time their status was known, e.g. the last time they were known to be alive. They contribute to the number of patients 'at risk' of the event up until this time point.
>
> *Reasons for censoring might include*
> 1. The event did not occur before the end of the study period
> 2. The subject died from an unrelated cause/accident
> 3. The subject moved away or withdrew from the study
>
> *Assumptions* 'Censored' individuals are assumed to have the same probability of the event in the period after they left the study as those subjects still remaining. This is likely to be true for reasons 1–2 but may not be true with 3. It is possible that subjects who moved away may be fitter and so have a lower probability of the event. Subjects who withdraw from a study might do so because of either treatment failure or treatment success, and so again they might be different from those who remain.

times, such as the range. For a randomized trial, these should be reported for each group separately. The report should state the reasons why subjects are lost to follow-up or censored, showing if possible that the reasons are unrelated to the probability of an event occurring (see box 11.1). In the Peripheral Vascular Disease study, most of the censored subjects had been recruited later in the study, and so had a shorter follow-up time. Note that, in a trial, patients may drop out if the treatment is not effective. These patients should be regarded as 'failures' and not as 'censored' observations.

11.1.2 Kaplan–Meier survival curves

Kaplan–Meier survival curves are a useful way of summarizing the survival, or time-to-event characteristics, of one or more groups of individuals and should be presented wherever possible. Box 11.3 gives useful tips on drawing these curves. Survival curves for peripheral vascular disease in patients with and without diabetes were produced in R using

---

Box 11.2 Using life tables in statistical packages   *HELPFUL TIPS*

Life tables
- Also known as actuarial analysis
- The life table method assumes that the event is known to occur within a time period rather than taking place at a specific time
- This method generally gives the same survival rates as Kaplan–Meier methods when survival times are not grouped
- In SPSS the user needs to set 'display time interval' to be the smallest time unit used, e.g. 1 month if survival is measured in months

Events taking place within first time period
- In Stata, **ltable** may be useful where events are recorded as taking place at the same time as recruitment, e.g. in the early pregnancy study time of miscarriage was reported in completed (whole) weeks. It was therefore possible for a woman to be recruited in the same week as she miscarried. In Stata, Kaplan–Meier methods would exclude these women, while the **ltable** command includes them.

---

the Kaplan–Meier method (figure 11.1). The graph shows that subjects with diabetes tended to die sooner than those without.

Kaplan–Meier survival curves are always shown as a series of steps, with the horizontal lines between steps indicating that the probability of survival remains constant between events. When describing or interpreting a curve, care should be taken not place too much emphasis on the right-hand side of the graph if the numbers at risk are small, or only a small proportion of the original sample remains in the study. The graph in figure 11.1 could be curtailed when the numbers of subjects at risk fell below 5 (see box 11.3). Where the

---

Box 11.3 Using Stata, SPSS, SAS, and R for survival analysis   *HELPFUL TIPS*

Terminating the graph when the number at risk is small
- Stata: Use 'tmax(#)' option, e.g. tmax(84) would truncate the curve in figure 11.1 at 84 months, where there are only 5 subjects at risk in the diabetic group
- SAS: Use 'MAXTIME=' option, e.g. 'MAXTIME=84'
- SPSS: Recode all cases with follow-up greater than the truncation point (84 months in this example) as censored for purposes of drawing the graph
- R: Use 'xlim=' argument for many plotting functions

Displaying numbers at risk
- Stata: Use 'atrisk' option to do this for every time point displayed. Note that, where there are many time points, as in the diabetes data, the result looks very cluttered.
- SAS: Use 'atrisk' option with the plot option

Displaying censored observations These are usually indicated by a tick on the survival curve but can be hidden if required.

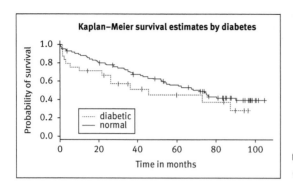

Figure 11.1 Kaplan–Meier curve (R)

number of subjects is large and they have been followed up for differing lengths of time, it may be wise to curtail the graph when only 10% of the original sample is still at risk.

The numbers at risk are displayed at regular time points, showing that the number at risk is much smaller in the diabetes group, especially in the right-hand portion of the graph. It may be useful to present the censored points on the graph, as shown by the vertical tick marks in figures 11.1 and 11.2. This indicates that most censoring took place towards the end of the study, most likely because subjects were still alive when the study ended.

11.1.3 Low event rates

If the event rates are less than 30% then the curves will be confined to the top third of the graph, and important differences in event rates may not be visible. Figure 11.3 shows

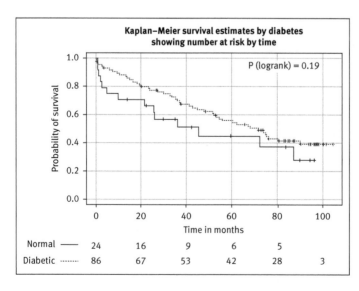

Figure 11.2 Kaplan–Meier curve with logrank test (R)

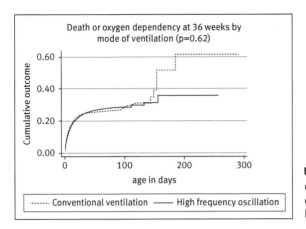

Death or oxygen dependency at 36 weeks by mode of ventilation (p=0.62)

.... Conventional ventilation ——— High frequency oscillation

Figure 11.3 Kaplan–Meier curve plotted upwards to show differences between groups that have low event rates (Stata)

a Kaplan–Meier curve for death or oxygen dependency at 36 weeks postmenstrual age and has been plotted with 1-survival rather than survival; hence, it has an upward shape. It shows that there is no real difference in survival between the two groups up to 150 days after which the curves begin to separate. However, the numbers at risk decreased to just 6% of the original total (49/797) at 150 day because few babies were being followed up after this. Hence beyond 150 days the precision is very poor and the graph could be curtailed at this point. For further discussion of presenting survival plots in clinical trials see Pocock et al. 2002.

11.2 Kaplan–Meier estimates of survival rates

Box 11.4 gives an example of the description of the Kaplan–Meier method for the methods and results sections of a paper. The survival rate at 5 years has been presented for each group with the 95% confidence interval. It is better to decide in advance which time point(s) to present. This may be consistent with convention, e.g. many cancer studies report five-year survival rates, although for cancers with poor survival a one-year rate may be more appropriate. The proportions should be calculated after taking censored observations into account, such as those produced by the Kaplan–Meier method.

Figure 11.4 shows the outputs from Stata, giving survival estimates at 12 and 60 months with 95% confidence intervals, and a logrank test comparing survival in the two groups.

11.3 The logrank test

It is possible to compare survival curves by comparing the survival at a particular point. However, this causes some difficulty since there are many different points that could be chosen and the choice is rather arbitrary. To test the difference in the curves at several points would lead to multiple testing and possible spurious significance. The logrank test avoids this problem by comparing the whole curve for each of the groups, and makes no assumptions about the shape of the survival curves provided they do not cross. If

> **Box 11.4 Presenting Kaplan–Meier analysis**
>
> ## Peripheral Vascular Disease study
>
> *Aim of study* To assess the long-term survival of patients with peripheral vascular disease (pvd) and to investigate the impact of the presence of risk factors on mortality.
>
> *Study design* Cohort study.
>
> *Patient population* Consecutive patients with pvd who were referred for angiography, and found to have angiographic evidence of pvd.
>
> *Aim of analysis* To compare survival rates in those with and without risk factors, including diabetes.
>
> ### Description
>
> *Methods section* Survival rates are expressed as the percentage surviving for 5 years, calculated using the Kaplan–Meier method. Kaplan–Meier curves comparing patients with and without diabetes are shown up to 7 years follow-up. The logrank test was used to test the difference between the survival curves.
>
> *Results section* One hundred and ten subjects were included in this analysis. Mean follow-up time of survivors was 6.1 years, range 14 days to 8.7 years. Thirty-five men and 26 women died. The Kaplan–Meier curve shows that patients with diabetes have lower survival rates (figure 11.2). The 5-year survival rate was 45%, 95% CI (23 to 65%) among those with diabetes and 56% (44 to 66%) among those without. The logrank test gave $P = 0.19$.
>
> For further information see Missouris CG, Kalaitzidis RG, Kerry SM, Cappuccio FP. Predictors of mortality on patients with peripheral vascular disease: a prospective follow-up study. *Br J Diabetes Vasc Dis* 2004; 4:196–200.

the curves do cross, the logrank test has low power to detect differences, i.e. the survival experiences may be still be different even though the test is not statistically significant. For example, in a cancer trial one group might experience early deaths due to drug toxicity but have better long-term survival. In that case we could not say that one drug has better or worse death rates *overall*; the different time periods need to be investigated separately.

The logrank test is summarized in box 11.5. A worked example of the test is given in Peacock and Peacock 2011 (chapter 8). Figure 11.4 shows the Stata output for this test. These results are included in the reporting of the analysis in box 11.4. Alternative approaches would be to include the estimated hazard ratio with its 95% CI (section 11.4), or to show error bars at regular points on the curve. The error bars could relate either to the standard error of the estimate of survival or to the confidence interval, but it is important to make clear which has been used. For a fuller discussion see Pocock et al. 2002. Note that, although we have only analysed two groups here, the Kaplan–Meier method and the logrank test can be used for three or more groups.

11.4 Cox regression

Previously, we have compared survival in two or more groups using the logrank test. We have also calculated estimates of survival at specific points to allow the curves to be directly

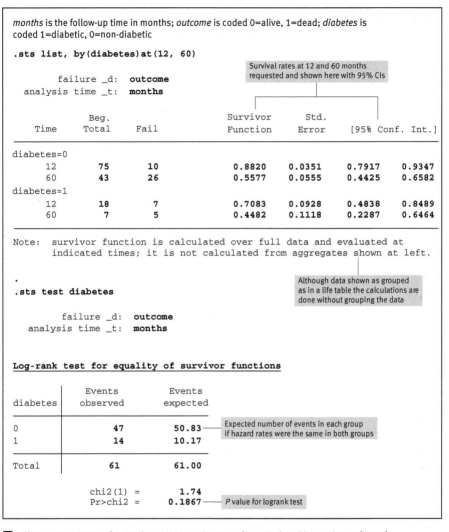

months is the follow-up time in months; outcome is coded 0=alive, 1=dead; diabetes is coded 1=diabetic, 0=non-diabetic

```
.sts list, by(diabetes)at(12, 60)
```

Survival rates at 12 and 60 months requested and shown here with 95% CIs

```
        failure _d:  outcome
   analysis time _t:  months

                 Beg.                    Survivor     Std.
    Time        Total    Fail            Function    Error    [95% Conf. Int.]

diabetes=0
      12          75      10              0.8820     0.0351    0.7917    0.9347
      60          43      26              0.5577     0.0555    0.4425    0.6582
diabetes=1
      12          18       7              0.7083     0.0928    0.4838    0.8489
      60           7       5              0.4482     0.1118    0.2287    0.6464
```

Note: survivor function is calculated over full data and evaluated at indicated times; it is not calculated from aggregates shown at left.

```
.
.sts test diabetes
```

Although data shown as grouped as in a life table the calculations are done without grouping the data

```
        failure _d:  outcome
   analysis time _t:  months
```

Log-rank test for equality of survivor functions

```
               Events        Events
   diabetes    observed      expected

   0               47          50.83
   1               14          10.17

   Total           61          61.00
```

Expected number of events in each group if hazard rates were the same in both groups

```
            chi2(1) =      1.74
            Pr>chi2 =    0.1867
```

P value for logrank test

Figure 11.4 Output for Kaplan–Meier estimates of survival and logrank test (Stata)

compared. However, it would be useful to have an overall measure of comparison of the survival experience of the groups. This can be done using the hazard ratio, which is calculated using the Cox proportional hazards model. The hazard ratio is the ratio of the probability or risk of an event occurring in one group compared to another, and the interpretation is similar to a relative risk. (The hazard ratio is sometimes referred to as a relative risk, but is more correctly called the hazard ratio.)

There are no assumptions about the shape of the survival curve, but the method assumes that the ratio of the probability of an event taking place in the two groups does not change over time. The simplest way to check this assumption is to see if the survival curves are approximately parallel. In small datasets there may be some crossing over if the curves are close together even when the assumption holds, but in this case there is unlikely to be a

Box 11.5 The logrank test
INFORMATION

Null hypothesis There is no tendency for survival to be shorter in one group than in the other.

Suitable for
- Analysing time to any event where each subject can have only one event. Survival times must be continuous or ordinal
- Two or more groups

Assumptions
- Subjects who are censored have the same probability of having the event as those fully followed up (see box 11.1)
- There is no tendency for one group to have better survival at early time points and worse survival at later time points. If this was not true the curves would diverge and might cross over each other.
- Note this is the same assumption as required by Cox regression, i.e. that the hazards, the probabilities of the event, are proportional (box 11.6)

Limitation Test of significance only.

Box 11.6 Cox proportional hazards models
INFORMATION

Cox regression model
- Used to obtain the ratio of the probability or risk of an event in two groups, called a 'hazard ratio'
- The hazard ratio may be interpreted as the relative risk of an event in the two groups
- Cox regression can be used to adjust the group effect for confounders or to test the effect of several possible predictor variables

Assumptions
- Subjects who are censored have the same probability of having the event as those fully followed up (box 11.1)
- The hazard ratio does not vary with time, i.e. the hazards are proportional to each other
- Large sample method: rule of thumb is that **at least 10 events per predictor variable** are required for estimates to be reliable (Peduzzi et al. 1995)
- Note that since not all subjects will experience the event, this will lead to a substantially larger sample size than 10 *subjects* per predictor

Simple check on the proportional hazards assumption
- Are the survival curves parallel?

If assumptions not met
- If the hazards are not proportional, consider treating the covariate as time-varying or stratify the analysis (we advise obtaining statistical input for these options)
- If the sample is too small for the rule of thumb above, consider whether it's possible and reasonable to use less covariates, or use an exact survival method

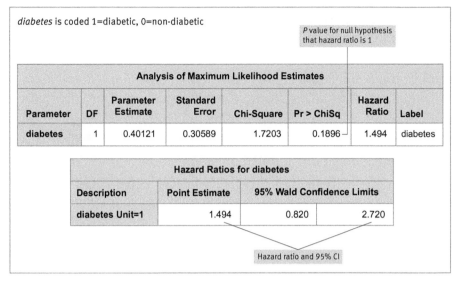

diabetes is coded 1=diabetic, 0=non-diabetic

P value for null hypothesis that hazard ratio is 1

		Analysis of Maximum Likelihood Estimates					
Parameter	DF	Parameter Estimate	Standard Error	Chi-Square	Pr > ChiSq	Hazard Ratio	Label
diabetes	1	0.40121	0.30589	1.7203	0.1896	1.494	diabetes

Hazard Ratios for diabetes		
Description	Point Estimate	95% Wald Confidence Limits
diabetes Unit=1	1.494	0.820 · 2.720

Hazard ratio and 95% CI

Figure 11.5 Output for Cox regression with one predictor available (SAS)

significant difference between the curves. If, on the other hand, curves do genuinely cross over then a single estimate of the ratio of risks is clearly meaningless and so great care is needed that the assumptions do hold.

Box 11.6 summarizes the method and its assumptions. For further discussion of methods to check the assumptions, see Bland 2015. We suggest that researchers seek the advice of a statistician when analysing survival data as it is a complex procedure to perform and interpret.

11.4.1 Presenting the results of single variable Cox regression

Figure 11.5 shows the output from SAS for the single variable Cox regression analysis. The output for this and figure 11.6 have been trimmed slightly to save space but the full versions are available on the web. The analysis is carried out on the logarithm of the hazard ratio. The coefficient therefore needs to be back-transformed using the exponential function to give the hazard ratio. Some packages report the hazard ratio by default (Stata), while others

---

Box 11.7 Presenting Cox regression with one predictor variable   *EXAMPLE*

Peripheral Vascular Disease study

(This adds to the analysis and description in box 11.4)

Methods section Cox regression was used to calculate the hazard ratio and 95% confidence interval.

Results section Patients with diabetes had shorter survival time than those without, but this was not significant (hazard ratio 1.49, 95% CI 0.82 to 2.72, $P = 0.19$).

diabetes is coded 1=diabetic, 0=non-diabetic
age70 is coded 1=age 70+, 0=age below 70

P value for hazard ratio for diabetics compared
to non-diabetics adjusted for age

Analysis of Maximum Likelihood Estimates							
Parameter	DF	Parameter Estimate	Standard Error	Chi-Square	Pr > ChiSq	Hazard Ratio	Label
diabetes	1	0.55504	0.31314	3.1417	0.0763	1.742	diabetes
age70	1	0.68321	0.26885	6.4576	0.0110	1.980	age70

Hazard Ratios for diabetes		
Description	Point Estimate	95% Wald Confidence Limits
diabetes Unit=1	1.742	0.943	3.218

Hazard Ratios for age70		
Description	Point Estimate	95% Wald Confidence Limits
age70 Unit=1	1.980	1.169	3.354

Hazard ratio for diabetics compared with
non-diabetics adjusted for age

Figure 11.6 Output for Cox regression with more than one predictor variable (SAS)

give both the coefficients on the log scale and its exponential, i.e. the hazard ratio (SAS, SPSS, R). Box 11.7 shows how the results of this Cox regression analysis can be presented as an addition to the analysis presented earlier in box 11.4.

11.4.2 Comment on the results

It was noted that age was significantly related to the risk of death and may be an important confounder in assessing the contribution of other risk factors. The diabetic subjects were younger than the non-diabetics, and so might be expected to have a lower death rate. The difference in age between the diabetics and non-diabetics might have reduced the estimated effect of diabetes on survival seen in the survival curves.

11.4.3 Extending the analysis

In section 11.4.2, Cox regression was used to perform an analysis with just one predictor variable (diabetes). However, Cox regression can be used to fit multifactorial models with several predictor variables and can therefore be used to estimate the hazard ratios after adjusting for other variables. The analysis was extended to adjust for age (see figure 11.6, SAS). The unadjusted and the adjusted hazard ratios are shown in the

---

Box 11.8 Presenting Cox regression analysis   *EXAMPLE*

Peripheral Vascular Disease study

Aim of study To assess the long-term survival of patients with peripheral vascular disease (pvd) and to investigate the impact of particular risk factors on mortality.

Study design Cohort study.

Patient population Consecutive patients with pvd who were referred for angiography and found to have angiographic evidence of pvd.

Aim of analysis To compare survival rates in those with and without particular risk factors, including diabetes.

Table **Survival rates and hazard ratios for risk factors of mortality in patients with peripheral vascular disease**

Risk factor		No. of deaths (%)	Percent. surviving 5 years (95% CI)	HR (95% CI)	HR (95% CI) adjusted for age
Age:	70+	37 (64)	38 (26, 51)	1.83 (1.09, 3.06)	
	<70	24 (46)	69 (54, 80)		
Diabetes:	Yes	14 (58)	45 (23, 65)	1.49 (0.82, 2.72)	1.74 (0.94, 3.22)
	No	47 (55)	56 (44, 66)		

Description

Methods section Survival rates are expressed as the percentage surviving for 5 years, calculated using the Kaplan–Meier method. Cox proportional hazards regression was used to calculate the hazard ratios and 95% confidence intervals for the risk factors. Age was treated as a covariate.

Results section One hundred and ten patients were included in this analysis. Mean follow-up time for survivors was 6.1 years, range 14 days to 8.7 years. Thirty-five men and 26 women died. The Kaplan–Meier curve shows that patients with diabetes had poorer survival (figure 11.2) but this was not significant ($P = 0.19$).

The increase in mortality risk was nearly two-fold in patients aged 70+ years compared to those under 70. After adjusting for age, patients with diabetes still had an increased risk of mortality compared to those without diabetes, but this was not statistically significant. Further adjustment for sex was made but had little effect on the hazard ratio (hazard ratio 1.70; 95% CI 0.96, 3.37, $P = 0.069$).

For further information see Missouris CG, Kalaitzidis RG, Kerry SM, Cappuccio FP. Predictors of mortality on patients with peripheral vascular disease: a prospective follow-up study. *Br J Diabetes Vasc Dis* 2004; 4:196–200.

---

table in box 11.8. The adjusted hazard ratio for diabetes is larger than the unadjusted ratio, but the confidence interval still crosses the null value of one. The Kaplan–Meier survival curves are not repeated here, but are referred to in the text and should be included, where possible, for the main comparison of interest. Note that it is possible to adjust Kaplan–Meier curves in Stata, which would show the curves to be further apart than in box 11.4. (Missouris et al. 2004).

**Box 11.9 Useful references to statistical details presented
in this chapter**   *INFORMATION*

Introductory accounts Bland 2015 (chapter 16); Peacock 2011 (chapters 8, 12); Altman 2000 (chapter 4)

Survival plots Pocock et al. 2002; Walker and Shostak 2010 (chapters 21, 22); Allison 2010 SAS (examples throughout); Maindonald and Braun 2010 (chapter 8)

Assumptions Bland 2015 (chapter 16); Peacock 2011 (chapters 8, 12)

When assumptions do not hold Bland 2015 (chapter 16)

Fuller accounts Collett 2003

Worked examples of the Kaplan–Meier methods Peacock 2011 (chapter 8); Bland 2015 (chapter 16)

11.5 Further reading

The references given in box 11.9 are those we have found particularly useful for the specific topics listed.

Box 11.10 Survival analysis   *CHAPTER SUMMARY*

♦ Survival methods are used to analyse time-to-event data. The outcome is not always death—it can be, for example, time to recurrence, time to miscarriage, time to conception, etc.

♦ Present the number of events, follow-up time, and variability in follow-up time

♦ Describe any censored observations and justify any assumptions made about them

♦ Survival curves should be shown, indicating censoring or numbers at risk

♦ Beware of imprecision in right-hand side of survival curve

♦ Estimate survival probabilities at a fixed time point, with 95% confidence intervals, using a method which takes into account censored observations (e.g. Kaplan–Meier)

♦ Beware of comparing survival at several points along the curves, unless there is a strong prior hypothesis, as this is multiple hypothesis testing and may lead to spurious significant results

♦ Use the logrank test to provide an overall comparison of two or more curves

♦ Present the hazard ratio with a 95% CI to estimate the difference in survival between two groups of interest. This can be calculated using Cox regression.

♦ Use Cox regression to adjust survival for several variables

♦ Check the assumptions for Cox regression hold

CHAPTER 12

Presenting a randomized controlled trial

12.1   **Introduction to the CONSORT statement** *173*

12.2   **The CONSORT checklist** *174*

12.3   **Intention-to-treat analysis** *189*

12.4   **Cluster randomized trials** *191*

12.5   **Reporting guidelines for other study designs** *193*

12.1 Introduction to the CONSORT statement

In the 1990s an international group of clinical trialists, statisticians, epidemiologists, and editors developed the CONSORT statement (**Con**solidated **S**tandards **of R**eporting Trials), to guide researchers on the reporting of randomized controlled trials (Begg et al. 1996). The CONSORT statement comprises a 25-item checklist and diagram with explanatory notes, and was revised and expanded in 2001 and 2010 (Schulz et al. 2010, Moher et al. 2010). Now CONSORT has been adopted by many biomedical editors as the standard for submissions to their journals, and the guidelines are readily available on the web (http://www.consort-statement.org). We summarize the rationale behind CONSORT in box 12.1.

The CONSORT checklist is shown in table 12.1. Detailed explanatory notes, with examples of good practice, are given on the CONSORT website and are well worth reading. The guidelines were designed for trials where individuals are randomly allocated to one of two or more treatment groups. However, the principles clearly apply to other more complex experimental designs as well.

In this chapter we will give examples in which the CONSORT statement is used to guide the presentation of statistical aspects of a two-group trial with individual randomization. The main example is from the UKOS trial that was published in 2002. This paper was reported according to the 2001 CONSORT guidelines, and a comment is given in the few cases where the 2010 guidelines require more information. Examples are also given from other published trials.

The same principles of reporting apply when presenting a trial in a longer document where space is less restricted and where the researcher is able to report in more detail than is possible in most journal articles. At the conclusion of the chapter we will briefly mention other designs, such as cluster designs, and summarize additional guidelines for reporting them.

Box 12.1 The CONSORT Statement   *INFORMATION*

Background

- Evidence-based medicine requires reliable scientific information about effective healthcare interventions
- A randomized controlled trial that is rigorously designed and carefully conducted and analysed provides the best evidence of the effectiveness of an intervention
- The quality of the design and reporting of randomized trials is known to be variable
- Flaws in design and reporting have been associated with biased and unreliable results

CONSORT (http://www.consort-statement.org)

- Consolidated Standards of Reporting Trials (revised 2010)
- 25-item checklist and flow-chart template, with accompanying explanatory notes
- Provides a common standard for reporting to guide researchers in presenting randomized trials
- Provides a framework for the critical review of randomized trials to facilitate valid decisions about healthcare practice

---

Since the original CONSORT statement for reporting trials was published, several extensions have been produced to cover particular situations. Those that are currently available are listed in box 12.2. Clusters trials are considered in more detail in section 12.4. Pragmatic trials (Eldridge 2010) are those that are designed to test the effectiveness of an intervention when used in the usual conditions of care. The pragmatic trials checklist gives specific guidance on the checklist items 2, 4, 5, 6, 7, 11, 13, and 21, which relate to the description of the eligibility criteria for the participants, the intervention, and the outcomes and the generalizability of the findings and so allow the reader to assess how far the intervention is applicable to a particular routine care situation.

12.2 **The CONSORT checklist**

In this chapter we focus attention on reporting items which relate to statistics and will refer back to previous sections in the book if a particular issue has been discussed before. We will indicate the specific CONSORT checklist items discussed in each paragraph.

12.2.1 **Title and abstract (checklist items 1a, b)**

The title of the paper and the abstract should indicate that the study is a randomized trial so that it gets indexed by electronic databases as a trial, and is thus accessible to other researchers performing electronic searches. In UKOS, the title did not mention 'trial' or 'randomized' and this would be required under the current 2010 guidelines, but it was clear from the abstract that this was a trial (box 12.3). We note that a later follow-up of the UKOS trial participants published in 2013 did include the phrase 'randomized trial' in the title (Zivanovic et al. 2014).

Table 12.1 CONSORT checklist (http://www.consort-statement.org) *INFORMATION*		
Section/Topic	**Item No.**	**Checklist item**
Title and Abstract	1a	Identification as a randomized trial in the title
	1b	Structured summary of trial design, methods, results, and conclusions (for specific guidance see CONSORT for abstracts)
Introduction		
Background and objectives	2a	Scientific background and explanation of rationale
	2b	Specific objectives or hypotheses
Methods		
Trial design	3a	Description of trial design (such as parallel, factorial) including allocation ratio
	3b	Important changes to methods after trial commencement (such as eligibility criteria), with reasons
Participants	4a	Eligibility criteria for participants
	4b	Settings and locations where the data were collected
Interventions	5	The interventions for each group with sufficient details to allow replication, including how and when they were actually administered
Outcomes	6a	Completely defined pre-specified primary and secondary outcome measures, including how and when they were assessed
	6b	Any changes to trial outcomes after the trial commenced, with reasons
Sample size	7a	How sample size was determined
	7b	When applicable, explanation of any interim analyses and stopping guidelines
Randomization		
Sequence generation	8a	Method used to generate the random allocation sequence
	8b	Type of randomization; details of any restriction (such as blocking and block size)
Allocation concealment mechanism	9	Mechanism used to implement the random allocation sequence (such as sequentially numbered containers), describing any steps taken to conceal the sequence until interventions were assigned
Implementation	10	Who generated the random allocation sequence, who enrolled participants, and who assigned participants to interventions
Blinding	11a	If done, who was blinded after assignment to interventions (for example, participants, care providers, those assessing outcomes) and how
	11b	If relevant, description of the similarity of interventions
Statistical methods	12a	Statistical methods used to compare groups for primary and secondary outcomes
	12b	Methods for additional analyses, such as subgroup analyses and adjusted analyses

Table 12.1 *continued*

Section/Topic	Item No.	Checklist item
Results		
Participant flow (a diagram is strongly recommended)	13a	For each group, the numbers of participants who were randomly assigned, received intended treatment, and were analysed for the primary outcome
	13b	For each group, losses and exclusions after randomization, together with reasons
Recruitment	14a	Dates defining the periods of recruitment and follow-up
	14b	Why the trial ended or was stopped
Baseline data	15	A table showing baseline demographic and clinical characteristics for each group
Numbers analysed	16	For each group, number of participants (denominator) included in each analysis and whether the analysis was by original assigned groups
Outcomes and estimation	17a	For each primary and secondary outcome, results for each group, and the estimated effect size and its precision (such as 95% confidence interval)
	17b	For binary outcomes, presentation of both absolute and relative effect sizes is recommended
Ancillary analyses	18	Results of any other analyses performed, including subgroup analyses and adjusted analyses, distinguishing pre-specified from exploratory
Harms	19	All-important harms or unintended effects in each group (for specific guidance see CONSORT for harms)
Discussion		
Limitations	20	Trial limitations, addressing sources of potential bias, imprecision, and, if relevant, multiplicity of analyses
Generalizability	21	Generalizability (external validity, applicability) of the trial findings
Interpretation	22	Interpretation consistent with results, balancing benefits and harms, and considering other relevant evidence
Other Information		
Registration	23	Registration number and name of trial registry
Protocol	24	Where the full trial protocol can be accessed, if available
Funding	25	Sources of funding and other support (such as supply of drugs), role of funders

Reproduced from *The BMJ*, CONSORT 2010 Statement: updated guidelines for reporting parallel group randomised trials, Kenneth F Schulz, Douglas G Altman, and David Moher, 340, copyright 2010, with permission from BMJ Publishing Group Ltd.

12.2.2 Trial design (checklist items 3a, b)

In keeping with the 2001 guidelines, the trial design was not explicitly described in the 2002 UKOS paper. However, the description very much implied that allocation is 1:1 and that the design is two parallel groups, so there is no real ambiguity.

> **Box 12.2 Extensions of the CONSORT Statement**   *INFORMATION*
>
> **Trial designs**
>
> ♦ Cluster trials
>   *Trials which randomize groups of individuals to interventions*
> ♦ Non-inferiority and equivalence trials
>   *Trials which aim to show one intervention is therapeutically similar to another*
> ♦ Pragmatic trials
>   *Trials which test whether an intervention works in routine care*
>
> **Interventions**
>
> ♦ Acupuncture interventions
> ♦ Herbal medicinal interventions
> ♦ Non-pharmacologic treatment interventions
>
> **Data**
>
> ♦ Abstracts
> ♦ CONSORT-PRO
>   *Guidance on reporting patient reported outcomes, whether primary or secondary outcomes*
> ♦ Harms
>
> Data from http://www.consort-statement.org/extensions

12.2.3 Participants (checklist items 4a, b)

A trial report should state the inclusion and exclusion criteria, and the settings and locations of the trial. These factors are important because they assist the interpretation of the trial results, and indicate the participant group to which the findings can be generalized. An example is shown in box 12.3. Note that there were eligibility criteria for the centres themselves, as well as inclusion criteria for the participants within the centres.

12.2.4 Intervention (checklist item 5)

In drug trials it is important to describe any steps taken to disguise a placebo. For example, a placebo-controlled trial of vitamin D supplementation described 'identical-looking pills containing vitamin D3, calcium carbonate, both, or placebo' (Rees et al. 2013). It may not be possible to blind (or mask) the intervention received in non-drug trials (see section 12.2.8).

In non-drug trials such as UKOS, where the intervention was a ventilator device, detailed explanation may be needed to describe adequately the different components of the intervention. For example, in a review of six trials of nurse-led hypertension clinics (Oakeshott et al. 2005), some trials had allowed the nurse to prescribe or recommend changes in drug treatment, while in others the emphasis was on healthy lifestyle advice. This highlights the need to provide full details of the intervention, and also to define what is meant by 'usual care'.

Box 12.3 Examples for CONSORT checklist items relating to the trial methods *EXAMPLE*

Item 1

Title

'High-frequency oscillatory ventilation for the prevention of chronic lung disease of prematurity'.

Allocation to intervention (Abstract)

'We randomly assigned preterm infants with a gestational age of 23 to 28 weeks to either conventional or high-frequency oscillatory ventilation. . .'

Item 4

Eligibility criteria

'Infants were eligible for the study if their gestational age was between 23 weeks and 28 weeks plus 6 days; if they were born in a participating centre; if they required endotracheal intubation from birth; and if they required ongoing intensive care. Infants were excluded if they had to be transferred to another hospital for intensive care shortly after birth or if they had a major congenital malformation.'

Settings and locations

'A total of 25 centres participated in the study—22 in the United Kingdom and 1 each in Australia, Ireland and Singapore. To ensure that each centre had adequate experience with high frequency oscillatory ventilation, we required participating centres to have used this type of ventilatory support in a minimum of 20 infants before the study began.'

Item 6

Outcomes

'The primary outcome measure was a composite of death or chronic lung disease (defined by a dependence on supplemental oxygen) at 36 weeks of postmenstrual age. Secondary outcome measures were age at death, age at hospital discharge, major abnormality on cranial ultrasonography, air leak, failure of treatment, failure on hearing testing, necrotising enterocolitis, patent ductus arteriosus requiring treatment, treatment with postnatal systemic corticosteroids, pulmonary haemorrhage, and retinopathy of prematurity.'

Item 7

Sample size

'A sample size of 800 to 1200 infants was needed, given the assumption that 30% of the study population would have a gestational age of 23 to 25 weeks and 70% would have a gestational age of 26 to 28 week and that the incidence of the primary outcome would be 75% for the lower-gestational-age group and 48% for the higher-gestational-age group. With a sample of this size, the study had 90% power (at a significance level 0.05), to detect a difference between treatment groups of 9 to 11 percentage points.'

Box 12.3 *continued*

Items 8–10

Randomization

'Infants were randomized in blocks of four to either conventional ventilation or high frequency oscillatory ventilation, with stratification according to gestational age (2 strata) and according to centre (25 strata).'

Item 12

Statistical methods

'An independent committee reviewed statistical analyses performed at 12 and 18 months after recruitment began and found no reason to stop the trial early. P values (*for the primary outcome*) were adjusted to preserve an overall level of significance as 0.05. For the secondary outcomes (both main effects and interactions), we used the Bonferroni method to correct for multiple testing, which resulted in the use of a P value of 0.004 to indicate significance. All reported P values are uncorrected unless otherwise stated. . . .'

'Unadjusted relative risks or hazard ratios, as appropriate, with 95% confidence intervals, were calculated to estimate the relative effect of high frequency oscillatory ventilation as compared with that of conventional ventilation for all outcomes. Logistic regression or Cox regression was used to investigate treatment effects with gestational age (23 to 25 weeks or 26 to 28 weeks) and location (United Kingdom and Ireland; Australia; or Singapore) as covariates. Interaction terms were fitted in the model in order to assess differences in treatment effects according to gestational age and location. Baseline variables with the potential to be important prognostic factors were identified in advance of the analysis. We decided to include them in the model only if a clinically important imbalance was observed. All statistical analyses were performed according to the intention-to-treat principle, with the use of Stata software.'

From *The New England Journal of Medicine*, Johnson A et al., High frequency oscillatory ventilation for the prevention of chronic lung disease of prematurity, 347, 9, p. 633. Copyright © 2002 Massachusetts Medical Society. Reprinted with permission from Massachusetts Medical Society.

It can be difficult to provide an adequate description of an intervention for a journal article. Box 12.4 gives some helpful tips about doing this, and box 12.5 gives an example from a trial of an intervention to increase physical activity in older adults (PACE-Lift). In pragmatic trials it is also important to report how the practitioners were selected to administer the intervention, and what training they received, for example, in trials of acupuncture or physical therapy (UK BEAM Trial Team 2004). For more guidance see the CONSORT extensions listed in box 12.2.

12.2.5 Outcomes (checklist items 6a, b)

It is important to report which outcome is pre-specified as the primary one, and then list any secondary outcomes. The primary outcome is the endpoint that will be used to determine

| Box 12.4 Describing interventions | *HELPFUL TIPS* |

- Identify the key components of the intervention
- Identify the key people involved in delivering the intervention
- Use a table to describe the main features of the key components
- Consider graphical methods to illustrate how the components work together and who delivers each:
  - *Cascade diagrams (Hooper et al. 2013) are useful to describe how the different personnel involved in a complex intervention work together*
  - *The method by Perera et al. 2007 describes the time line for the different trial activities.*
  - *A useful example is given in Pinto et al. 2014, which uses both approaches to describe their intervention.*
- Publish the protocol and include more detailed information in the protocol, which can then be referred to in the main trial report
- Add 'on-line appendices' to the main paper
- Develop and use training manuals and appropriate patient material

if there is a real difference between the two interventions, and is used in the sample size calculations. Secondary outcomes are other outcomes of interest, and may include adverse effects of the interventions. For each outcome, especially the primary outcome, the type of data should be clear. For example, is it a measurement, a score, or a category? This information helps the reader to understand the statistical analysis, and it aids the interpretation of the findings.

The example shows the primary and secondary outcomes from UKOS (box 12.3). Care was taken to define any terms that are potentially ambiguous or uncommon, such as 'chronic lung disease'. The primary outcome is a yes/no (binary) variable. No changes were made to the trial outcomes after the trial began but it clearly would be important to report this if it had happened.

12.2.6 Sample size (checklist items 7a, b)

The presentation of sample size follows the guidelines given in chapter 3. It is important to give enough information to allow the calculations to be checked by reviewers and other researchers. The information required includes: power, significance level (usually two-sided in superiority trials, as described here), the difference between treatment groups that can be detected with the target number of participants (effect size), and standard deviation (continuous outcomes). If the sample size calculations have made allowance for attrition during the trial, this should be described.

The clinically meaningful difference in treatments is not only important for the sample size calculations, but also to aid interpretation of the observed difference in treatment groups. Some studies report expected differences which are very big and seem unlikely.

Box 12.5 Describing an intervention   *EXAMPLE*

PACE-Lift trial

Table from the main trial paper (extract)

Components	What was provided
Pedometer	Yamax Digi-Walker SW-200 model
Accelerometer	Actigraph GT3X+ (LLC)
Practice nurse physical activity (PA) consultations	Four individually tailored PA consultations with the Practice nurse Participants could be seen individually or as a couple
Patient handbook	Patient handbook to support 12-week walking plan
Walking/PA plan	Individual walking plane
PA diary	PA diary to record weekly PA for 12 weeks. Step counts and walks

More information was given:

1. In the paper in a 3rd column of the table to describe the components in detail
2. In the protocol which contained a description of each component mapped to a theoretical model for behaviour change
3. In the patients' handbook and diary that were available online from the publisher's website

This can arise if the researcher's baseline (control group) estimate is too low, and/or the anticipated estimate (intervention group) is too high. Sometimes, large 'expected' treatment differences result from the researcher having a fixed and small available sample size, and so the researcher has worked backwards to calculate the difference which this sample size could detect. In this situation, the trial is likely to produce a smaller difference in treatment outcome than expected. This will be non-significant and therefore the trial will be inconclusive.

The sample size statement from UKOS is shown in box 12.3. Two things are worth noting here. First, a range was given for the target sample size. This represented minimum and maximum feasible numbers which could be recruited in the time available and therefore translated into a range for the difference to be detected. The clinicians felt this was reasonable since defining the clinically meaningful difference involves judgement. Second, two values were given for the estimated proportion with the primary outcome—one in the lower gestational-age infants, and the other in the higher gestational-age infants. The calculations were presented in this way because it is common to present outcome rates for lower and higher gestational-age infants separately, and this therefore showed clearly how the overall figures were obtained.

Where trials have interim analyses for data monitoring purposes, it is important to state how many times the committee met and what steps were taken to deal with multiple testing of outcomes. If a complex stopping rule was used, this should be described. The UKOS paper reported the data monitoring information with the other statistical analysis (box 12.3, item 12). It is not always necessary to follow the checklist order if information fits better elsewhere. The important thing is to include all of the information clearly.

12.2.7 Randomization (checklist items 8–10)

The CONSORT checklist requires fairly detailed information on the randomization process. This includes reporting how the random sequence was generated, confirming that it was truly random, and stating who allocated participants to their groups. For example, a telephone or a web-based service could be used. It should be clear who has recruited the participants since it is important to be able to demonstrate that the randomization was separate from the recruitment, and that the recruitment of participants could not be biased by knowledge of the allocation sequence, a process known as 'allocation concealment'.

If unrestricted simple randomization is used, this should be stated. If randomization was restricted using blocks and/or strata, this should be described, stating the block size and listing the stratification variables.

The statement shown in box 12.3 comes from the published paper and is noticeably brief; although full details were submitted to the journal, these were omitted due to lack of space. Box 12.6 shows the details of randomization from the PACE-Lift trial.

The checklist in table 12.1 assumes patients are individually randomized to intervention groups. If this is not the case, then the unit of randomization should be stated. Section 12.4 describes the key features of cluster randomized designs where groups of individuals are randomized to intervention groups.

12.2.8 Blinding (checklist items 11a, b)

Blinding is important to avoid biased assessment and should be reported when it is used. The term 'masking' is a preferable to 'blinding' since it better describes what is happening,

---

Box 12.6 Describing a trial randomization   *EXAMPLE*

PACE-Lift trial

'Participants with adequate baseline accelerometer data were randomised using the Nottingham Clinical Trials Unit internet randomisation service. Randomisation was at household level to avoid couple contamination. Block randomisation was used within practice with random sized blocks, varying between 4 and 6, and 1:1 allocation ratio, to ensure group balance and an even nurse workload. Participants were informed by telephone of their group allocation. Researchers were not blind to intervention status at assessments.'

i.e. the researcher is aiming to conceal the allocation—but both terms are still used. Researchers should report if the participants were masked to the treatment allocation, since knowledge of the treatment is known to affect response. Also, it is important to report whether those assessing the outcome were masked to the treatment allocated since knowledge of the treatment received may subconsciously or consciously affect the assessment of all outcomes, with the probable exception of death.

Trials are not always conducted masked and in some cases masking is impossible, for example, when the interventions are two different technologies. In UKOS the intervention was one of two types of ventilator which could not be concealed from the clinician. The participants in UKOS were infants and so would be unaware of the type of intervention. Wherever possible, assessments were done by independent observers who were unaware of the ventilator used.

When designing a trial, it may be possible to choose the more objective methods of measurement from a set of possible alternatives. For example, the use of automatic blood pressure measuring devices may be less prone to observer bias than a mercury sphygmomanometer. It is important to report these design features since this increases the validity of the data.

12.2.9 Statistical methods (checklist items 12a, b)

This section should document the type of analysis performed to compare the primary outcome between the two groups. Unless it is obvious, any assumptions inherent in the methods should be justified. The researcher should describe the method used for any adjusted analyses, including the choice of variables to adjust for. Any subgroup analyses should also be described. Where adjustment was made for baseline imbalance, this should be described and justified. Any adjustment for multiple testing should be described. The researcher should say whether analyses were performed according to the intention to treat and, if not, then this should be justified (see section 12.3.1). It is helpful to state the statistical program used for the analysis.

The UKOS statement in box 12.3 includes details of most of these points, in particular, the methods used to adjust for multiple testing, methods for testing subgroup effects, and the strategy for dealing with imbalance in baseline variables.

12.2.10 Participant flow and recruitment details (checklist items 13–14)

It is important to provide a complete audit trail of a trial so that all participants are accounted for. Details of all eligible participants should be given, with reasons for non-recruitment, where available. Numbers of, and reasons for, post-randomization losses should be documented. A diagram is often the best way to show the flow of participants from recruitment to analysis. Figure 12.1 shows the template available on the CONSORT website, from which a Word version can be downloaded.

The UKOS participant flow diagram is shown in figure 12.2. The diagram makes clear how many infants were eligible, and how many of these were recruited, plus the reasons for non-recruitment. Since consent and randomization sometimes happened before birth, some infants were later found to be ineligible and were excluded. Further losses occurred due to withdrawals for various reasons. All infants were accounted for, showing finally the number of infants included in the analysis of the primary outcome.

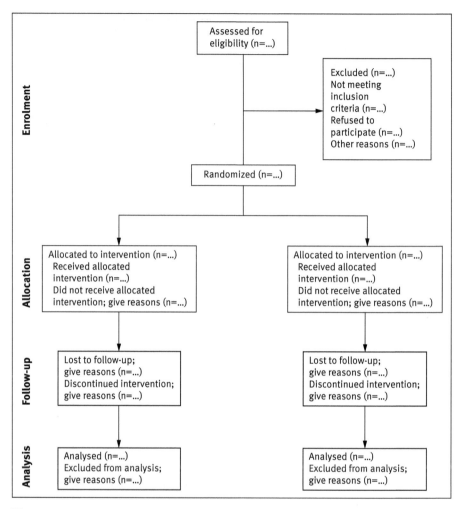

Figure 12.1 Template for the CONSORT flowchart

It is also important to report the dates of the trial, since the date of publication of a paper may not be a good indicator of when the trial took place. Box 12.3 shows how the recruitment process can be described in the text. Note that any protocol deviations should be reported in the original randomization groups.

12.2.11 Baseline data (checklist item 15)

It is important to present baseline data in a trial for two reasons. The first is to show the characteristics of the group so that readers can judge how applicable the trial results are to a specific individual. The second is to confirm that the two randomized groups are balanced for key prognostic variables. If the participants have been allocated to the two groups at random, then any imbalance between the groups must be due to chance alone, unless the randomization process was faulty.

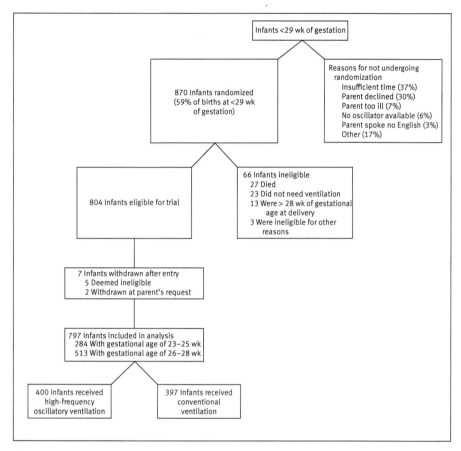

Figure 12.2 Diagram to show participant flow in a randomized controlled trial (example)

From *The New England Journal of Medicine*, Johnson A et al., High frequency oscillatory ventilation for the prevention of chronic lung disease of prematurity, 347, 9, p. 633. Copyright © 2002 Massachusetts Medical Society. Reprinted with permission from Massachusetts Medical Society.

Sometimes researchers use a significance test to compare the two groups at baseline (pre-randomization) and to report a *P* value for this. We do not recommend this practice since, if participants have been allocated randomly to the two groups, any differences between the groups must be due to chance alone. Testing against chance makes no sense.

Baseline data in the two trial groups can be reported in a similar way to data for a single group (chapter 4). The table of baseline characteristics needs to include the following for each group: number of subjects, mean and standard deviation for continuous data, and perhaps the median and range if the data are skewed, and the proportion or percentage, with numerator and denominator, for categorical data.

Box 12.7 shows an extract from one of the two tables of baseline variables from UKOS, with a sentence describing these findings. Baseline data for mothers and infants separately were reported separately.

UKOS Study

Baseline characteristics of the mother (extract)

Characteristic	HFOV	CV
	N=364	**N=353**
Age (yr) mean (SD)	29 (6.4)	29 (6.1)
Race: no/total (%)		
White	290/363 (80)	276/353 (78)
Black	35/363 (10)	31/353 (9)
Other	38/363 (10)	46/353 (13)
Pre-existing or pregnancy-induced diabetes	11/364 (3)	7/351 (2)
Smoking in pregnancy: no/total (%)	95/334 (28)	86/321 (27)
Caesarean section		
After labour	75/364 (21)	64/353 (18)
Without labour	134/364 (37)	125/353 (35)

HFOV: High frequency oscillatory ventilation; CV: conventional ventilation.
The total numbers relate to mothers not infants, as some births were multiple.

Description

The two treatment groups were well balanced for maternal characteristics.

Data from Johnson AH, Peacock JL, Greenough A, Marlow N, Limb ES, Marston L et al. High-frequency oscillatory ventilation for the prevention of chronic lung disease of prematurity. *N Engl J Med* 2002; 347:633–642.

Note that deficiencies in the patients' medical notes led to incomplete data for some variables.

12.2.12 Outcome data (checklist item 17)

Since the primary outcome is the endpoint used to assess the effectiveness of the study interventions, it is essential that it is prominently reported in the text and in the abstract, whatever the results may show. All specified secondary outcomes should similarly be reported, whether significant or not. For all outcomes the effect size should be given with a measure of precision, such as a confidence interval, except where this is not possible, for example, when using rank-based methods. If there is space, the P value could be given as well. If rank-based tests are used that only give a P value, it is useful to report summary statistics by group such as median and interquartile range.

These guidelines should be followed whether or not the primary or secondary outcome is statistically significant. Confidence intervals are especially important where a finding is not statistically significant, since it will indicate whether or not the findings suggest that a clinically important difference may exist.

It is quite common to present a confidence interval for each group separately. This is not helpful, since the main interest is the difference between the groups and that cannot

---

Box 12.8 Example of a CONSORT checklist item relating to outcomes   *EXAMPLE*

UKOS Study

Primary and secondary outcomes at 36 weeks postmenstrual age (extract)

Outcome	HFOV	CV	Relative risk (HFOV/CV) (95% CI)
Primary outcome: no/total (%)			
All infants	265/400 (66)	268/397 (68)	0.98 (0.89 to 1.08)
Dead	100/400 (25)	105/397 (26)	
Alive, with chronic lung disease	165/400 (41)	163/397 (41)	
Alive, without chronic lung disease	135/400 (34)	129/397 (32)	
Secondary outcomes: no/total (%)			
Failure of treatment	41/400 (10)	41/397 (10)	0.99 (0.66 to 1.50)
Major cerebral abnormality	54/393 (14)	75/393 (19)	0.72 (0.52 to 0.99)
Air leak	64/399 (16)	72/395 (18)	0.88 (0.65 to 1.20)
Pulmonary haemorrhage	44/395 (11)	55/390 (14)	0.79 (0.55 to 1.14)

HFOV: High-frequency oscillatory ventilation; CV: conventional ventilation

Description

'The composite primary outcome of death or chronic lung disease (defined as dependence on supplementary oxygen) at 36 weeks of postmenstrual age) occurred in 66% of infants assigned to high-frequency oscillatory ventilation and 68% of those assigned to conventional ventilation (P=0.71). Similar proportions of infants died (25% of those receiving high-frequency oscillatory ventilation vs 26% of those receiving conventional ventilation) or had chronic lung disease (41% in each group). The proportions of infants with each of the specified secondary outcomes were also similar in the two groups. In particular, criteria for treatment failure were met in 10% of the infants in each group.'

Data from Johnson AH, Peacock JL, Greenough A, Marlow N, Limb ES, Marston L et al. High-frequency oscillatory ventilation for the prevention of chronic lung disease of prematurity. *N Engl J Med* 2002; 347:633–642.

---

be easily deduced from separate intervals. Also, reporting two separate intervals plus an interval for the difference clutters the results.

Box 12.8 shows an extract of the outcome data for UKOS, and the wording used to describe the findings. The primary outcome was binary, and the difference between the two ventilation groups was expressed as a relative risk with a 95% confidence interval. The difference between the two treatment groups was small—two percentage points—and the interval spanned 1.0 and was clearly not significant. Had the difference been statistically significant, it may have been useful to report the number needed to treat (see section 12.3.2) as well as the relative risk.

Note that the secondary outcome, major cerebral abnormality, has a 95% confidence interval that excludes 1.00 and so indicates significance at the 0.05 level. However, for secondary outcomes, the trial calculated a modified cut-off for significance (0.004) to avoid getting spurious significant results simply due to testing multiple variables. This finding was commented on in the discussion section of the paper. Note that if a Bonferroni correction is used for a set of significance tests, then the overall analysis is testing a composite of all the separate hypotheses (see Bland and Altman 1995 for further details).

12.2.13 Reporting harms data (checklist item 19)

Adverse event data are often poorly collected and reported compared to the reporting of efficacy outcomes. This can make it difficult to interpret the net benefit of one treatment compared to another. The CONSORT for harms statement (http://www.consort-statement.org/extensions) helps guide the reporting of harms. Cornelius et al. 2013 discusses some of the issues and makes suggestions for ways to improve the collection and reporting of harms data in pain studies.

12.2.14 Interpretation and presentation of a non-significant result (checklist item 20)

It is important to interpret 'not significant' correctly when describing the difference between the two treatment groups. If the trial is powered to detect a small clinically important difference, then a non-significant finding will indicate that there is no important difference between the groups. However, it does not mean that there is evidence for no difference at all, and it is essential to present the estimated difference between the groups, and a confidence interval.

If the result is non-significant and the trial is small, then it is entirely possible that an important difference does exist but that the trial is simply too small to demonstrate this conclusively. It is always wrong to interpret non-significance as meaning that there is 'no difference' between the treatments. Instead, the results should be reported as inconclusive, and the interpretation should focus on the range of true effect values represented by the confidence interval.

Non-significant results should always be reported, in large and small trials. This allows the reader to interpret the findings in the light of other studies, and perhaps pool results with those of others in a meta-analysis, to obtain a more precise overall estimate.

12.2.15 Ancillary analyses (checklist item 18)

Researchers sometimes perform other analyses which are not the stated primary or secondary outcome analyses. Subgroup analyses fall into this category. Effects in subgroups should always be tested by fitting an interaction term in the model. For example, in UKOS, the effect of treatment in the two gestational-age groups was tested by fitting an interaction term in the model and not by looking at the two groups separately. It can be useful to present subgroup analyses graphically in a similar way to a forest plot (section 13.4.10). Harris et al. 2015 presented a forest plot for their subgroup analysis for the PACE-Lift trial (figure 12.3).

Subgroup analyses are sometimes conducted in a post hoc, data-driven fashion, i.e. the idea of doing the analysis comes from looking at the data. This is problematic because if a large effect is observed and then tested it is clearly more likely to be statistically significant than an observed small effect. If post hoc analyses are done for exploratory reasons, the findings should be reported tentatively and any findings interpreted with caution. Chapter 13 discusses this issue further in the context of meta-analyses (see table 13.2).

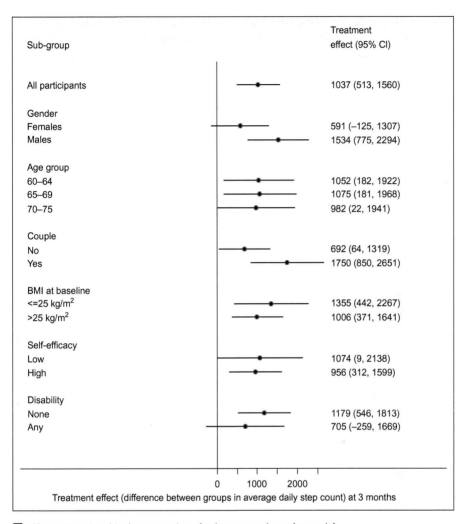

12.3 **Intention-to-treat analysis**

12.3.1 **Introduction**

When subjects are randomized, the two groups should be comparable with respect to base-line characteristics. If any subjects are excluded after randomization then this comparability will be compromised. It is therefore recommended that an intention-to-treat analysis

---

**Box 12.9 Example of intention to treat and numbers needed
to treat (NNT)**   *EXAMPLE*

Nicotine inhaler trial

Aim of study To see if oral nicotine inhalers lead to long-term reduction in smoking.

Design Double blind, randomized, placebo-controlled trial.

Setting Two university hospital pulmonary clinics in Switzerland.

Participants Four hundred healthy volunteers willing to reduce their smoking but
unable or unwilling to stop smoking immediately.

Intention to treat analysis All patients were analysed according to original allocation.
Patients who withdrew or were lost to follow-up were assumed to have continued
smoking.

Results 152/200 participants in the placebo group and 166/200 in the control group
completed four months of follow-up.

52 (26%) subjects in active group stopped smoking.

18 (9%) subjects in the placebo group stopped smoking.

Risk difference was 0.17 (95% CI: 0.10 to 0.24)

$$\text{Number needed to treat} = 1/\left(\text{Risk difference}\right)$$
$$= 5.9 \ \left(95\% \ \text{CI } 4.1 \text{ to } 10.3\right)$$

Data from Bolliger CT, Zellweger JP, Danielsson T, van B, X, Robidou A, Westin A et al. Smoking reduction with oral
nicotine inhalers: double blind, randomised clinical trial of efficacy and safety. *BMJ* 2000; 321:329–333

---

is carried out where all subjects are analysed according to the groups to which they were
originally allocated (section 12.2.9).

However, full application of intention to treat is only possible when complete outcome
data are available for all subjects (Hollis and Campbell 1999). In many trials, subjects will
have missing observations and these may not be a random sample of all subjects. It may
be that patients who do not perceive any benefit from the intervention withdraw from the
trial. In smoking cessation trials it is common practice to assume that patients who drop
out or do not give samples have continued to smoke (Bolliger et al. 2000; box 12.9). Such
an approach would not be suitable for all trials, especially those with continuous outcomes
(Hollis and Campbell 1999). It is therefore important to describe clearly what steps have
been taken to investigate any potential influence of missing responses.

Where patients have swapped treatment groups, either by dropping out of active treatment or being given a different treatment, intention-to-treat analysis will tend to underestimate the treatment benefit. This may not be desirable in an equivalence trial and may be
a reason for not carrying out an intention-to-treat analysis.

Box 12.10 Number needed to treat (NNT)   *SUMMARY*

♦ Used with binary outcomes

♦ Number needed to treat is the reciprocal of the risk difference (box 7.9)

♦ Calculate the risk difference and 95% confidence interval then take reciprocal of values

♦ Lowest possible value is 1 (negative values can be considered as the numbers needed to harm)

♦ Highest possible value is infinity (∞)

♦ If confidence interval for risk difference spans 0, e.g. $-p_L$ to p_U, then NNT can be written as $-\infty$ to $-1/p_L$, $1/p_U$ to ∞. It should not be written as $-1/p_L$ to $1/p_U$ (Bland 2015)

♦ NNT should only be used as an additional descriptive summary of the results and not as the main presentation of the outcome

---

12.3.2 Number needed to treat

The number needed to treat is the number of patients that would need to receive the new treatment in order to achieve one more success than on the old treatment. It is applicable only to binary outcomes, and the main features are presented in box 12.10. It is the reciprocal of the risk difference, which needs to be calculated first, along with its 95% confidence interval. An example is shown in box 12.9.

If the results are not statistically significant, then the presentation is problematic, as the confidence interval is not continuous and needs to be presented in two parts. For more details see Peacock and Peacock 2011 (chapter 10) and for a fuller discussion see Bland 2015 (chapter 8).

12.4 Cluster randomized trials

Cluster randomized trials are trials where groups of individuals, the clusters, are jointly allocated to an intervention so that all individuals within a cluster receive the same intervention. Hence, the cluster is the unit of randomization. Cluster trials are commonly used in primary care research, where it may be more practical to assign a whole general practice to the same intervention rather than to allocate individuals separately within a practice. Other units of randomization may be seen, for instance hospital wards, schools, whole communities such as villages in developing countries, time periods such as weeks, or airline flights.

Randomizing clusters rather than individuals has consequences for the required sample size and the statistical analysis of a trial, and therefore affects the presentation of a trial.

The required sample size will be greater when clusters are randomized because of the inter-dependence between individuals within each cluster. The level of increase in sample size depends on the size and number of clusters and the degree of inter-dependence between individuals in the clusters. We summarize these points in box 12.11. Methods for

---

Box 12.11 Cluster trials   *INFORMATION*

- Cluster trials randomly allocate *groups* of individuals, such as general practices or families or areas, to receive the same intervention
- Individuals in clusters are not independent—they are more similar to each other than to individuals in other clusters. This non-independence affects sample size calculations and statistical analysis
- The intraclass correlation coefficient measures the degree of correlation between individuals within clusters, and is used in sample size calculations
- Cluster trials tend to need more subjects than individually randomized trials, never less
- Cluster trials have a number of clusters and a number of individuals within the clusters. This two-level structure must be taken into account in the statistical analysis.
- Ignoring clustering in sample-size calculations leads to underpowered studies
- Ignoring clustering in analysis leads to P values that are too small and confidence intervals that are too narrow
- Reporting full details of the cluster trial design and analysis is essential for other researchers to be able to interpret the findings

---

Box 12.12 Extension to the CONSORT statement for cluster trials   *INFORMATION*

- Make clear in title that the trial is clustered
- Report the reasons for choosing a cluster design and define the cluster clearly
- Describe how participants within clusters are identified and recruited, and the steps taken to avoid selection bias
- Report how the effects of clustering were used in the sample-size calculations, including the value of the intraclass correlation coefficient (ICC) used, the number of clusters, and the number of subjects per cluster
- Report how clustering was allowed for in the analysis
- Give a flowchart of both clusters and individuals from recruitment to analysis
- Present baseline group data for clusters and for individuals
- Report the ICC for the primary outcome of the trial

For full details of the checklist and explanation see http://www.consort-statement.org/extensions

For a full explanation of cluster trials see Eldridge and Kerry's practical guidebook (Eldridge and Kerry 2012)

Data from http://www.consort-statement.org/extensions

> **Box 12.13 Selected other reporting guidelines**   *INFORMATION*
>
> **Selected reporting guidelines for trials and other designs** (http://www. equator-network.org)
> - **SPIRIT** (Standard Protocol Items: Recommendations for Interventional Trials): for trial protocols
> - **PRISMA** (Preferred Reporting Items for Systematic Reviews and Meta-Analyses)
> - **STROBE** (Strengthening the Reporting of Observational Studies in Epidemiology)
> - **STARD**(Standards for Reporting of Diagnostic Accuracy)

sample size calculations are shown in Kerry and Bland 1998a, and a simple way of analysing cluster randomized trials using summary measures for each cluster is described in Kerry and Bland 1998b.

Campbell et al. 2012 proposed an extension to the CONSORT statement specifically for cluster trials. Like the general CONSORT statement, the statement for cluster trials provides explanations and examples of good practice, the main points of which are summarized in box 12.12. Researchers conducting and reporting cluster trials will find the full document very helpful (available on http://www.consort-statement.org). For a fuller discussion of cluster trials, see Eldridge and Kerry 2012. As most cluster trials are pragmatic, and non-pharmacologic interventions are common, the book contains a combined version of the three CONSORT extension statements with explanations.

12.4.1 Recruitment bias

In cluster randomized trials, extra care needs to be taken in reporting how the participants within the clusters were identified and recruited, whether this was before or after the allocation of the clusters to the intervention groups, and whether the person recruiting the participant was blind to the treatment allocation. For fuller discussion see Eldridge and Kerry 2012 or Puffer et al. 2003. Kerry et al. 2005b gives an example of steps taken to reduce recruitment bias in a health education trial in rural Ghana, where whole villages were randomized to an intervention or control programme.

12.5 Reporting guidelines for other study designs

Further reporting guidelines for many interventional and observational studies are available via the EQUATOR (Enhancing the **Qu**ality and **T**ransparency **o**f Health **R**esearch) website (http://www.equator-network.org). Some of the guidelines that are most commonly seen and used are listed in box 12.13; one in particular, PRISMA (**P**referred **R**eporting **I**tems for **S**ystematic Reviews and Meta-Analyses), is illustrated in chapter 13.

Box 12.14 Presenting a randomized controlled trial   *CHAPTER SUMMARY*

Follow CONSORT guidelines for reporting randomized controlled trials. In particular:

- Ensure study is clearly reported as a randomized controlled trial so it gets indexed as a trial for other users to find in electronic searches
- Show a flow chart from recruitment to analysis to account for all participants
- Describe sample size calculations in detail
- Describe randomization process and any blinding in detail
- Describe the statistical methods including any adjustment of P values for multiple testing and any variables that have been adjusted for
- Distinguish between planned and unplanned analyses
- Report the primary outcome prominently, whether significant or not
- Report all secondary outcomes whether significant or not
- For all outcomes, give an effect size, and whenever possible also give a measure of precision (95% CI)
- Don't assume that 'not statistically significant' means 'there is no difference' — look at the effect size and the width of the confidence interval
- Follow CONSORT cluster guidelines if unit of randomization is a cluster
- See CONSORT extension for other trial designs and EQUATOR to access other guidelines for other designs and issues

---

CHAPTER 13

Presenting a meta-analysis

13.1   **Introduction to systematic reviews and meta-analysis** *195*

13.2   **Statistics and meta-analysis** *200*

13.3   **The PRISMA statement** *200*

13.4   **Reviewing meta-analyses** *216*

13.5   **Further reading** *217*

13.1 Introduction to systematic reviews and meta-analysis

Meta-analysis is a statistical technique that combines the results of several independent studies that have examined the same research question. It is based on a systematic review of the evidence relating to the question of interest and aims to gain an overall view of the evidence. The pooling of data from multiple studies provides estimates that are more precise than those obtained from the original individual studies. Early meta-analyses were in perinatal medicine in the 1980s, where researchers sought to pool evidence from all available clinical trials to inform clinical practice. This led to the establishment of the (now) Cochrane Collaboration, which promotes the systematic review and meta-analysis of health evidence in all clinical areas (http://www.cochrane.org). Since the early meta-analyses of clinical trials, meta-analysis methods and practice have expanded to cover a wide range of quantitative study designs (box 13.1).

13.1.1 Defining the research question

Defining a good research question is key to a good systematic review, and needs careful thought as the researcher has no control over the design of the individual studies which will be included. Most meta-analyses use study-level data so the researcher will be deciding whether or not to include the whole study rather than individual participants in the analysis. There may be small differences in inclusion criteria between studies but if the majority of subjects are similar it will be possible to include more studies and hence more data if we are not too restrictive. Consequently, research questions tend to be broader in meta-analyses than in primary research studies.

A helpful way to define the research question is using the PICOS method described in box 13.2. The letters refer to the Population, Intervention, Comparator, Outcomes, and Study design. The letters PICO were initially designed for randomized trials but the same principle can be used for observational studies comparing risk factors if we think of the 'I' as Indicating a risk factor. Defining the elements of PICOS makes it easier to define the search terms and assess the eligibility of studies.

Box 13.1 Introduction to meta-analysis   *INFORMATION*

What is it?

♦ Meta-analysis is a statistical analysis that combines results from individual studies that examine the same research question. It is based on a review of all available evidence.

♦ All findings on a topic are pooled to gain an overall view and so this increases statistical power compared to the power for individual studies

♦ Meta-analysis may be carried out with aggregate study level data or individual patient level data (see box 13.4)

Bias in meta-analyses

♦ **Publication bias** may arise if any studies are excluded, for example because they are unpublished or not in the public domain or perhaps published in a foreign language. It is the most commonly seen form of study selection bias.

♦ **Outcome reporting bias** arises due to researchers selectively reporting some outcomes and omitting others. For example, researchers sometimes only report statistically significant outcomes and ignore non-significant ones.

♦ **Design bias:** Other forms of bias may arise from methodological flaws in the original studies, such as failure to conceal treatment allocation from researchers and/or participants.

♦ Selection bias, outcome-reporting bias, and design bias are commonly associated with **inflated effect sizes**.

Types of studies for meta-analysis

♦ Many meta-analyses pool data from randomized controlled trials but, increasingly, meta-analysis techniques are used for other designs such as cohort and case/control studies, diagnostic studies, and prevalence studies.

Box 13.3 gives an example of PICOS from a systematic review of home blood pressure monitoring. In this example it was important to state the definition of the comparator group precisely as in some trials patients monitored their blood pressure in both groups but in only one group were these readings used by clinicians to guide treatment decisions. Whether or not these studies should be included depends on the precise research question. In the review Bray et al. 2010 the authors were asking the pragmatic question, does asking patients to take their own blood pressure encourage better blood pressure control? In order to answer this question it is important that patients in the control group are not being asked to take their own blood pressure. Some trials were excluded because they did not measure blood pressure as an outcome, instead using patient compliance with medication.

13.1.2 Aggregate data versus individual patient data meta-analyses

Meta-analysis can either be carried out on study-level summary data or using individual patient data from a number of studies. The former method is the most common and allows the meta-analysis to be carried out without the co-operation of the original authors,

Box 13.2 Defining a research question using PICOS *INFORMATION*

Population

Consider who is to be included in the analysis. Common issues are:

- Children, adults or older adults
- Primary vs secondary care
- Health care system
- Diagnosis and severity of disease

Intervention—for randomized trials

What is the intervention? Common issues are:

- Specific drug or all drugs in drug class
- Different routes of administration
- Different dosage
- Whether to allow studies with concomitant interventions

Indicator (Risk factor)—for observational studies

What is the risk factor and how is it measured?

- Different exposures
- Timing of exposure (ever, past, current)
- Length of time

Comparator for randomized trials

This is likely to be one or more of:

- Placebo
- Usual care or standard treatment
- An alternative treatment not usually given as standard care

Comparator for observational studies

May be useful to consider:

- Never or not currently exposed
- Low levels of exposure or none

Outcomes

How will the effect be measured?

- Patient-orientated outcomes or clinical outcomes
- Intermediate or surrogate endpoints
- Disease specific or all-cause outcome
- Timing of outcome
- Composite endpoints may have slightly different definitions in different studies

---

Box 13.2 *continued*

Study design

♦ Most interventions will include randomized controlled trials (RCTs) only but, where there are few RCTs for practical or ethical reasons, non-randomized trials or cohort studies may be included

♦ Observational studies are likely to be either cohort studies, case-control studies, or diagnostic studies

---

Box 13.3 Example of PICOS   *EXAMPLE*

Example: Systematic review of home blood pressure monitoring

'The objectives were to determine the effect of self-monitoring of blood pressure in adults on blood pressure and blood pressure control, compared to usual care (no self-monitoring of BP). The outcomes used were office and ambulatory systolic and diastolic blood pressure, and number of patients meeting office target blood pressure.'

'RCTs were eligible if the intervention tested included self-measurement of BP without medical professional input, if usual care did not include patient self-monitoring, and if a blood pressure outcome measure was available that had been taken independently of the self-measurement (either systolic or diastolic office pressure or ambulatory monitoring (mean day-time ambulatory pressure)).

Non-randomized designs were excluded.'

In these two statements the complete PICOS is described.

Population Adults

Intervention Self-measurement of BP without medical professional input

Comparator Usual care which did not include patient self-monitoring

Outcomes Blood pressure taken independently of the self-measurement

Study design Randomized trials

Reproduced from: Does self-monitoring reduce blood pressure? Meta-analysis with meta-regression of randomized controlled trials, Bray EP, Holder R, Mant J, and McManus RJ., Annals of Medicine, 2010; 42:371–386, reprinted by permission of the publisher (Taylor & Francis Ltd, http://www.tandfonline.com) http://www.informaworld.com

---

although they may be contacted if data are missing. Individual Patient Data (IPD) meta-analyses are much more time consuming and difficult to carry out because of the difficulty in obtaining the data and collating data, which are stored in different formats using different coding schemes (box 13.4).

> **Box 13.4 Aggregate data versus individual patient data**
> **meta-analysis** *INFORMATION*
>
> **Aggregate data meta-analyses**
>
> - These use study-level summary data such as the overall relative risk or mean difference using published studies or other analysed datasets
> - The study-level data are relatively easy to obtain if the data are in the public domain such as peer-reviewed journal articles
> - Study-level data can only be combined when they have common outcomes and, even then, subtle differences in how an outcome is measured may affect the ability to pool estimates
> - The original study authors need not be contacted unless data are missing
>
> **Individual patient data (IPD) meta-analyses**
>
> - These use the raw data from the individual studies to provide pooled estimates for chosen outcomes
> - They allow more flexibility than meta-analyses that rely on aggregated data, as common outcomes can be derived for all studies from the raw data
> - Unlike aggregated data meta-analyses, IPD meta-analyses allow individual patient characteristics to be incorporated into the analyses so that differences between studies can be adjusted for and/or subgroup effects explored
> - IPD meta-analyses are not straightforward since it can be difficult to obtain the raw data from all relevant studies if researchers are not contactable, the raw data are lost, and/or researchers are not be willing or permitted to share their data
> - Combining the datasets, allowing for differences in coding, format of data, etc., is very time-consuming

13.1.3 Bias in meta-analysis

A meta-analysis provides an unbiased answer to a research question if all evidence is obtained from rigorously conducted studies, and all studies are available and pooled. The main types of bias that are commonly found in meta-analyses are study selection bias and outcome-reporting bias (box 13.1). Selection bias occurs when some studies are not available or are difficult to obtain. Specifically, there is a tendency for studies which fail to show a significant effect to remain unpublished, be published in more obscure and/or non-English language journals, or have their publication delayed. This is also known publication bias. Outcome-reporting bias occurs when researchers do not present results on all outcomes analysed. Again, this can happen because some results are not statistically significant and so considered uninteresting. Other forms of bias occur due to methodological flaws in the design or conduct of studies such as inadequate concealment of the treatment allocation. Most biases in meta-analysis lead to an inflation of the pooled estimate and so this is a serious problem as seemingly effective interventions may not in fact work. The introduction of reporting guidelines is therefore an important step to ensure that the presentation of systematic reviews and meta-analyses is thorough and transparent. In this way the meta-analysis design and conduct, and any shortcomings, are clear and can be taken into consideration by other researchers when they interpret the meta-analysis results. For more details about presenting bias in individual studies see section 13.3.7 and for bias in selection of studies see section 13.3.11.

13.2 Statistics and meta-analysis

Box 13.5 outlines the main statistical terminology seen in meta-analyses of randomized controlled trials. Pooled estimates are usually obtained by taking a weighted average of the individual study estimates, which gives greater weight to more precise studies. The actual weighting depends on whether fixed or random effects are used.

13.2.1 Heterogeneity between studies

The baseline assumption when conducting a meta-analysis is that the studies being pooled are homogeneous and that they all represent the same underlying study population and effect. Any observed variability between the studies would be simply due to random sampling from the same population. If the observed variability is greater than would be expected by random sampling alone, there is evidence for statistical heterogeneity (see box 13.5). This might be because the effect is different in different populations. The type of analysis used is different in these two cases, with a random effects model being used where there is evidence of heterogeneity, and a fixed effects model otherwise. The interpretation of the estimate, its 95% confidence interval, and its *P* value are, broadly speaking, the same for fixed and random effects meta-analyses.

13.3 The PRISMA statement

In chapter 12 we described the CONSORT reporting guidelines for clinical trials and here describe the reporting guidelines for systematic reviews and meta-analyses. PRISMA (Preferred Reporting Items for Systematic Reviews and Meta-Analyses) is a 27-item checklist and flowchart template, and provides a common standard of reporting meta-analyses (Moher et al. 2009). It replaces the 'QUOROM' statement (box 13.6). The PRISMA guidelines have been widely adopted by journals in the same way as the CONSORT statement for randomized trials has been.

In this chapter we give an example of a published meta-analysis that includes the UKOS study data shown in previous chapters and we show how it conforms to PRISMA. We also give examples from other meta-analyses to illustrate particular features. The full set of items in the PRISMA checklist can be seen in table 13.1.

13.3.1 Introduction to the examples

As in chapter 12, we will focus our attention to the reporting of items that relate to statistics. The meta-analyses used as an example use IPD from each study rather than the summary measures from each published study (Cools et al. 2010). The aim of the meta-analysis was to assess the effectiveness of high-frequency oscillatory ventilation (HFOV) versus

---

Box 13.5 Statistical methods and terms used in meta-analysis   *INFORMATION*

Analyses

◆ **Pooled estimates** are obtained using statistical analyses that provide a weighted average of the individual results. The weighting means that less precise studies contribute proportionately less than more precise ones. Outcomes can be binary, such as risk difference, relative risk, or odds ratio, or continuous, such as a mean difference.

◆ **Fixed effects analyses** are the default and assume that the studies are homogeneous, i.e. that they all have the same underlying outcome value

◆ **Random effects analyses** do not assume that contributing studies have the same underlying outcome value. The calculation of the overall value allows for this heterogeneity.

◆ The degree of **heterogeneity** between studies can be quantified using a statistic called I^2, which has a 0–100% scale. The presence of heterogeneity can be examined using a statistical test based on the chi-squared distribution.

Analysis for IPD

◆ **One-stage model:** In this approach all the data are analysed using one statistical model that takes into account the structure of the data, i.e. it comes from a number of different studies

◆ **Two-stage model:** In this approach each study is analysed separately but using common definitions and methods and then pooled in the same way as for aggregate data meta-analysis

Presenting results

◆ **Risk of bias** in the individual studies can be presented graphically or in a table, distinguishing between clear evidence of high or low risk of bias from studies where risk is unclear (see figure 13.2)

◆ The results of meta-analyses are often displayed graphically in a **forest plot**. This shows the results for each individual study with a 95% CI, and shows the overall pooled value (see figures 13.3 and 13.4 for examples). Results are sometimes given in a table as well.

◆ Potential selection bias is often explored graphically, e.g. using a **funnel plot** (see figure 13.5)

◆ It is good practice to report the **study characteristics** for each study to help interpret the results (see table 13.2)

---

conventional ventilation (CV) in all studies conducted in very preterm infants. UKOS was included in the review. A previous Cochrane review by the same lead authors, using the reported summary data from each study, had been conducted and found no evidence for any differences using published data. However, the Cochrane review was unable to look at subgroups, for example, defined by gestational age, since not all studies reported

---

Box 13.6 The PRISMA Statement   *INFORMATION*

PRISMA (http://www.prisma-statement.org)
- ◆ Preferred Reporting Items for Systematic Reviews and Meta-Analyses
- ◆ 27-item checklist and flow-chart template with accompanying explanatory notes
- ◆ Provides a common standard of reporting to guide researchers in presenting meta-analyses
- ◆ Provides a framework for the critical review of meta-analyses to facilitate valid decisions about health care practice
- ◆ Replaces the previously used QUOROM statement
- ◆ One of a growing number of reporting guidelines that can be located on the EQUATOR website (http://www.equator-network.org)

---

gestational age subgroup results and those that did defined the subgroups slightly differently. By using the raw data as in the current IPD meta-analysis, it was possible to define subgroups in the same way for all studies.

In general, there are many distinct advantages to conducting an IPD meta-analysis but it is rarely seen due to the substantial practical difficulties in accessing all the raw data. From a reporting and interpretational point of view, there are few differences between an aggregate data meta-analysis (the type usually seen) and IPD, and PRISMA covers both. Where there are differences we comment in the text.

13.3.2 Title (checklist item 1)

The title should identify the paper as a systematic review or meta-analysis, as it does here (box 13.7). This ensures that it is correctly indexed by electronic databases and is accessible to other researchers. Here, the title also states that this meta-analysis is based on individual patients' data.

13.3.3 Rationale and objectives (checklist items 3, 4)

It is important to set the scene and explain why the review was needed and what the specific objectives were. Here, the objectives were to plug the gap in evidence about whether HFOV might have different effects according to the babies' characteristics, or the clinical setting. This is important information that is directly applicable to clinical practice.

Because this paper reported on an IPD meta-analysis, it was important to give a brief account of how this came about. Hence, the paper reported that the IPD meta-analysis was organized by a collaborative group (PreVILIG (Prevention of Ventilator Induced Lung Injury collaborative Group)) who developed and agreed the meta-analysis protocol.

13.3.4 Protocol and registration (checklist item 5)

A meta-analysis is a research study in its own right and requires a protocol. PRISMA requires that the protocol is accessible to readers of the paper so that they can verify that the searches, analyses, and subgroup analyses were pre-planned. For this meta-analysis this was particularly important since the objectives included planned subgroup analyses.

Table 13.1 PRISMA checklist (https://www.prisma-statement.org)   *INFORMATION*

Section/topic	Item no.	Checklist item
Title		
Title	1	Identify the report as a systematic review, meta-analysis, or both.
Abstract		
Structured summary	2	Provide a structured summary including, as applicable: background; objectives; data sources; study eligibility criteria, participants, and interventions; study appraisal and synthesis methods; results; limitations; conclusions and implications of key findings; systematic review registration number.
Introduction		
Rationale	3	Describe the rationale for the review in the context of what is already known.
Objectives	4	Provide an explicit statement of questions being addressed with reference to participants, interventions, comparisons, outcomes, and study design (PICOS).
Methods		
Protocol and registration	5	Indicate if a review protocol exists, if and where it can be accessed (e.g., Web address), and, if available, provide registration information including registration number.
Eligibility criteria	6	Specify study characteristics (e.g., PICOS, length of follow-up) and report characteristics (e.g., years considered, language, publication status) used as criteria for eligibility, giving rationale.
Information sources	7	Describe all information sources (e.g., databases with dates of coverage, contact with study authors to identify additional studies) in the search and date last searched.
Search	8	Present full electronic search strategy for at least one database, including any limits used, such that it could be repeated.
Study selection	9	State the process for selecting studies (i.e., screening, eligibility, included in systematic review, and, if applicable, included in the meta-analysis).
Data collection process	10	Describe method of data extraction from reports (e.g., piloted forms, independently, in duplicate) and any processes for obtaining and confirming data from investigators.
Data items	11	List and define all variables for which data were sought (e.g., PICOS, funding sources) and any assumptions and simplifications made
Risk of bias in individual studies	12	Describe methods used for assessing risk of bias of individual studies (including specification of whether this was done at the study or outcome level), and how this information is to be used in any data synthesis.
Summary measures	13	State the principal summary measures (e.g., risk ratio, difference in means).

Table 13.1 *continued*

Section/topic	Item no.	Checklist item
Synthesis of results	14	Describe the methods of handling data and combining results of studies, if done, including measures of consistency (e.g., I^2) for each meta-analysis.
Risk of bias across studies	15	Specify any assessment of risk of bias that may affect the cumulative evidence (e.g., publication bias, selective reporting within studies).
Additional analyses	16	Describe methods of additional analyses (e.g., sensitivity or subgroup analyses, meta-regression), if done, indicating which were pre-specified.
RESULTS		
Study selection	17	Give numbers of studies screened, assessed for eligibility, and included in the review, with reasons for exclusions at each stage, ideally with a flow diagram.
Study characteristics	18	For each study, present characteristics for which data were extracted (e.g., study size, PICOS, follow-up period) and provide the citations.
Risk of bias within studies	19	Present data on risk of bias of each study and, if available, any outcome level assessment (see item 12).
Results of individual studies	20	For all outcomes considered (benefits or harms), present, for each study: (a) simple summary data for each intervention group (b) effect estimates and confidence intervals, ideally with a forest plot.
Synthesis of results	21	Present results of each meta-analysis done, including confidence intervals and measures of consistency.
Risk of bias across studies	22	Present results of any assessment of risk of bias across studies (see Item 15).
Additional analysis	23	Give results of additional analyses, if done (e.g., sensitivity or subgroup analyses, meta-regression [see Item 16]).
DISCUSSION		
Summary of evidence	24	Summarize the main findings including the strength of evidence for each main outcome; consider their relevance to key groups (e.g., healthcare providers, users, and policy makers).
Limitations	25	Discuss limitations at study and outcome level (e.g., risk of bias), and at review-level (e.g., incomplete retrieval of identified research, reporting bias).
Conclusions	26	Provide a general interpretation of the results in the context of other evidence, and implications for future research.
FUNDING		
Funding	27	Describe sources of funding for the systematic review and other support (e.g., supply of data); role of funders for the systematic review.

Reproduced from *The BMJ*, The PRISMA statement for reporting systematic reviews and metaanalyses of studies that evaluate healthcare interventions: explanation and elaboration, Alessandro Liberati et al., 339, copyright 2009, with permission from BMJ Publishing Group Ltd.

PreVILIG Study

Item 1

Title

'Elective high frequency oscillatory versus conventional ventilation in preterm infants: a systematic review and meta-analysis of individual patients' data'

Items 3, 4

Introduction: rationale and objectives

'. . .important questions about the use of HFOV in preterm infants remain unanswered, including whether some preterm infants benefit more or less from HFOV than others and whether the effect of HFOV is modified by factors such as the type of high-frequency ventilator and the time of initiation of ventilation. . . . The Prevention of Ventilator Induced Lung Injury Collaborative Group (PreVILIG collaboration) was therefore formed with investigators of the randomised controlled trials to compare elective HFOV with conventional ventilation in preterm infants with respiratory failure, and a protocol was developed to undertake a systematic review with meta-analysis of individual patients' data.'

Item 5

Protocol and registration

'The protocol of this study has been published (Cools et al 2009) but is outlined here. . ..'

Item 6

Eligibility criteria

'Studies were included if preterm infants (<35 weeks' gestational age) with respiratory insufficiency necessitating mechanical ventilation were randomly assigned to elective HFOV or conventional ventilation—deemed elective if used as the main method of ventilation early in the course of disease. Trials entering babies after conventional ventilation that was deemed to have failed rescue were excluded.'

Items 7

Information sources, search and study selection

'We searched the most recent update of the Cochrane review of aggregate data (November, 2006), Medline, Embase, the Cochrane Controlled Trials Register (CENTRAL, Cochrane Library Issue 4, 2008), and the Oxford Database of Perinatal Trials using the MeSH terms "high-frequency ventilation" and "infant, premature". We searched for reports written in any language from 2006, until January, 2009 (figure 1).

Box 13.7 *continued*

We asked experts in the field to identify any ongoing or unpublished trials, although no studies were identified with this strategy.'

Item 9
Study selection

As for item 6.

Item 10

Data collection process

'For all trials with the original individual patients' data available, we requested anonymised data about patient baseline characteristics (17 items), experimental intervention (four items), control intervention (six items), co-interventions (seven items), and outcome measures (16 items) for every randomly assigned infant (web appendix pp 1–2).'

Item 11

Data items

'The pre-specified primary outcomes were death or bronchopulmonary dysplasia (defined as receipt of supplemental oxygen at 36 weeks' postmenstrual age, although the physiological requirement of supplemental oxygen, as tested by oxygen challenge, was not noted in any of the trials); death or severe brain injury (defined as grade 3 or 4 intraventricular haemorrhage, 17 cystic periventricular leucomalacia, or both, on ultrasound); and death or bronchopulmonary dysplasia at 36 weeks' postmenstrual age or severe brain injury. In all trials, deaths were included up to discharge home of the infant.

The pre-specified secondary outcomes were death before discharge; bronchopulmonary dysplasia at 36 weeks' postmenstrual age in survivors; grade 3 or 4 intraventricular haemorrhage; cystic periventricular leucomalacia; gross pulmonary air leak (defined as presence of pneumothorax, pneumomediastinum, or pneumopericardium, or a combination thereof); any pulmonary air leak (defined as presence of gross pulmonary air leak or pulmonary interstitial emphysema, or both); postnatal and postmenstrual age at final extubation; total number of days on mechanical ventilation; postnatal and postmenstrual age at last day of treatment with continuous positive airway pressure; postnatal and postmenstrual age at last day of treatment with oxygen; retinopathy of prematurity stage 2 or more; 18 patent ductus arteriosus requiring treatment; patent ductus arteriosus requiring surgical ligation; crossover from assigned to alternative ventilation method because of treatment failure; and postnatal age at discharge from neonatal intensive care unit.'

Item 12

Risk of bias

'We assessed risk of bias through analysis of the adequacy of random sequence generation, allocation concealment, blinding of outcome assessment (for

Box 13.7 *continued*

intraventricular hemorrhage, periventricular leucomalacia, and pulmonary air leak), and completeness of follow-up data. Full details of the risk of bias assessment are published in the updated Cochrane review (Cochrane Database Syst Rev 2009; **3:** CD000104).'

Items 13–14
Summary measures, synthesis of results

'A two-stage approach was used for the main analyses: for a specific outcome the effect estimate (relative risk and 95% CI) was calculated for each trial separately and subsequently combined across trials to calculate a summary estimate. A fixed-effect model was used. The presence of heterogeneity of recorded treatment effects between trials was tested with the chi-squared test for heterogeneity and the I^2 statistic, which expresses the proportion of heterogeneity that cannot be explained by chance.

Heterogeneity was deemed significant when P was less than 0.05 or I^2 was more than 50%. A random-effects model was used in all analyses to test the robustness of the results to the choice of the statistical model. In case of significant heterogeneity, results of the random-effects model are noted.'

Item 16
Additional analyses

'To explore treatment effects by patient characteristics, subgroup analyses were pre-specified on the basis of gestation at delivery, birthweight for gestation, initial lung disease severity (oxygenation index at trial entry; calculated by mean airway pressure [cm H2O]×fractional inspired oxygen concentration [FiO2]×100÷partial arterial oxygen tension [mm Hg]), antenatal treatment with corticosteroids, postnatal age at randomisation, and period of exposure to conventional ventilation before initiation of HFOV (time between intubation and study entry). Subgroup analyses added post hoc were sex of the infant, presence of chorioamnionitis, and timing of first dose of exogenous surfactant from study entry.

To explore effects by trial characteristics, pre-specified subgroup analyses were planned by high-frequency ventilator type (SensorMedics 3100A, CareFusion, San Diego, CA, USA vs other oscillators vs flow interrupters) and by ventilation strategy both for HFOV (optimal lung volume strategy or not) and for conventional ventilation (lung protective ventilation strategy or not).'

Reprinted from *The Lancet*, 375, 9731, Cools F, Askie L, Offriga M, Asselin JM, Calvert SA, Courtney SE et al., Elective high-frequency oscillatory ventilation versus conventional ventilation in preterm infants: a meta-analysis of individual patient data, pp. 2082–2091. Copyright 2010, with permission from Elsevier

The pre-specification of these in the published protocol provided both a clear plan and boundaries for the analyses that were to take place (Cools et al. 2009). It was also useful for the meta-analysis authors to be able to refer to the published protocol when replying to journal article reviewers who requested further subgroup analyses that had not be

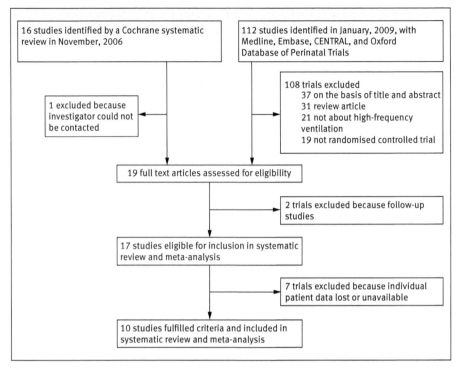

⬚ **Figure 13.1** Flow diagram for PreVILIG meta-analysis

Reprinted from *The Lancet*, 375, 9731, Cools F, Askie L, Offriga M, Asselin JM, Calvert SA, Courtney SE et al., Elective high-frequency oscillatory ventilation versus conventional ventilation in preterm infants: a meta-analysis of individual patient data, pp. 2082–2091. Copyright 2010, with permission from Elsevier

pre-specified. Having the protocol allowed the PreVILIG authors to be able to report these further analyses as clearly post-hoc.

13.3.5 Eligibility criteria, study selection, and information sources (checklist items 6, 7, 9, 17)

It is important to state the criteria for inclusion of the studies to enable readers to determine which group(s) of patients the results apply to. Information needed includes the characteristics of the patients, the interventions, the outcomes, and the study design. It is also necessary to document how the studies that were included were found—such as which databases were searched and whether any supplementary searches were conducted such as here, where experts in the field were consulted.

Figure 13.1 shows the process of identifying studies in a flow diagram with the numbers of studies identified and assessed at all stages through to the final set of eligible studies.

13.3.6 Data collection (checklist items 10, 11)

In an aggregate data meta-analysis, the data are obtained from published reports, most often published papers. The data are usually reported in a variety of formats in the original papers and so a carefully designed data collection form is needed. It is good practice for two independent researchers in the meta-analysis team to extract data separately and then to compare and have a pre-planned strategy to reach consensus if they disagree. This process should be described when reporting the meta-analysis.

In the IPD meta-analysis, uniformity of reporting is not an issue since the original pre-processed patient records are used, although of course the required data need to have been actually recorded by the original study researchers. The important thing to document for IPD meta-analyses is which particular variables were requested and obtained, as shown for this item in box 13.7. Additionally, for an IPD meta-analysis, it is necessary to state the outcomes that will be computed from the raw data. These are detailed against item 11.

13.3.7 Risk of bias in individual studies (checklist items 12, 20)

In this IDP meta-analysis, the quality of the studies was generally high as all contributing studies had attempted to conceal the randomization process. However, the interventions could not be blinded as this is not possible with these modes of ventilation. Bias can be avoided by blind assessment of outcomes where possible, such as having an independent reviewer to assess babies' scans and x-rays. This was done in UKOS. However, the lack of blindness in general could be associated with bias regarding the use of co-interventions and the ascertainment of outcomes, such as duration of mechanical ventilation and oxygen therapy.

Figure 13.2 gives an example of a graphical display of risk of bias from a meta-analysis of randomized trials of interventions to prevent weight gain in pregnancy. This graph differentiates studies where the information was unclear from those where the methods indicated a high risk of bias. Lack of clarity in the original article may be due to the space constraints of the journal rather than because the studies were not high quality. An example of this is in box 12.2, where some information was not included in the main UKOS paper.

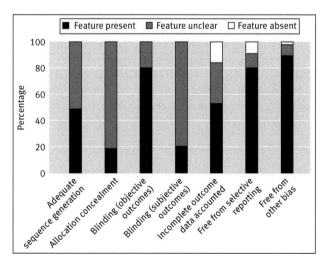

Figure 13.2 Example of risk of bias for trials included in a systematic review

Reproduced from *The BMJ*, Thangaratinam et al; 344:e2088 © 2012 with permission from BMJ Publishing Group Ltd.

13.3.8 Summary measures and additional analyses (checklist items 13–14, 16)

Meta-analyses that use aggregated data calculate a summary measure such as a pooled relative risk or odds ratio for binary outcomes, or a pooled mean difference for continuous outcomes. These need to be specified along with the type of model used (fixed or random effects) plus a description of how heterogeneity was assessed and, if present, dealt with.

In IPD meta-analyses, a common approach, and the one used in the PreVILIG study is to first calculate the summary outcomes for each study separately using the agreed common definitions applied to the raw data. Second, these are pooled across studies. This is known as a two-stage process (box 13.5). The second-stage analysis is the same as the analysis that is done for an aggregated data meta-analysis.

Note that a sensitivity analysis approach was used to compare results when fixed versus random effects models were fitted to check how much the model assumptions affected the results.

The *additional items* section in PRISMA documents the pre-planned subgroup analyses. This was particularly important here as exploring subgroups was the main reason for undertaking this IPD meta-analysis.

13.3.9 Study characteristics (checklist items 17, 18)

The flow diagram in figure 13.1 shows how the search strategy led to the final 17 studies, of which 7 could not be included because individual patient data was either lost or unavailable. The paper reports that the 10/17 studies with available data included 89% of randomized patients.

Table 13.2 shows how the characteristics of the ten included studies can be reported. The table only shows 3/10 studies, referred to as Moriette, Courtney, UKOS, due to lack of space, and reports first trial design characteristics, including the number of centres, the number of participants, and the type of machine used in the two trial arms (for high-frequency oscillatory or conventional ventilation). Second, patient characteristics are reported, including neonatal factors (gestational age, infant sex, singleton/multiple birth, time to randomization) and clinical factors (use of surfactant, corticosteroids, time to intubate the newborn baby). These factors were important to help the interpretation of the individual study results and the pooled results. Note that the studies were similar for most characteristics shown.

13.3.10 Results of individual studies (checklist items 20, 21)

Meta-analysis results are frequently presented as a forest plot only since this shows all the main features in one graph. Figure 13.3 shows a forest plot for the main outcomes in the PreVILIG IPD meta-analysis. The forest plot gives results for a composite binary outcome: death, or bronchopulmonary dysplasia (bpd) or severe adverse neurological events. Each study is given on a single line, with the main data in numbers as well as an overall relative risk depicted by a solid square with a 95% confidence interval indicated by a horizontal line. The sizes of the solid squares are proportionate to the size of the study so that the largest study, UKOS, has the biggest square. The overall pooled relative risk (RR) is shown by a solid diamond below the individual values. The width of the diamond depicts its 95% confidence interval (CI). The pooled RR is close to 1 (0.98) and the 95% CI is

Table 13.2	Examples for PRISMA checklist items relating to study characteristics		*EXAMPLE*

PreVILIG study

Item 18

Characteristics of included studies (Note only 3/10 studies, Moriette, Courtney, UKOS, are shown, due to lack of space)

Studies	Moriette	Courtney	UKOS
Trial design characteristics			
Number of centres	10	26	25
Number of participants	273	482	797
Type of HFOV	Dufour-OHF1	SensorMedics 3100A	SLE-2000HFO SensorMedics 3100A Drager Babylog 8000
Mode of conventional ventilation	SIMV	SIMV	SIMV or IPPV
Patient characteristics			
Mean (SD) gestation at birth (weeks)	27.2 (1.4)	26.1 (1.6)	26.1 (1.5)
Male infants	159 (58%)	260 (54%)	428 (54%)
Infants from multiple birth	81 (30%)	120 (25%)	190 (24%)
Surfactant therapy	273 (100%)	482 (100%)	769 (97%)
Median (IQR) time to intubation (min)	3 (2–5)	3 (1–8)	2 (1–4)
Median (IQR) time to randomization (min)144 (92–196)	166 (118–206)	<60	
Antenatal corticosteroids**	146 (54%)	443 (92%)	727 (92%)

**Any antenatal treatment with corticosteroids, irrespective of the timing to delivery.
HFOV: high-frequency oscillatory ventilation; IMV: intermittent mandatory ventilation; IPPV: intermittent positive pressure ventilation; IQR: interquartile range; SD: standard deviation; SIMV: synchronized intermittent mandatory ventilation; UKOS: UK Oscillation Study.
For further information see Cools F, Askie L, Offriga M, Asselin JM, Calvert SA, Courtney SE et al. Elective high- frequency oscillatory ventilation versus conventional ventilation in preterm infants: a meta- analysis of individual patient data. *Lancet* 2010; 375:2082–2091.

narrow and crosses 1, and so the RR is not statistically significant ($P = 0.61$). The test for statistical heterogeneity is not significant, with a low I^2 ($P = 0.28$, $I^2 = 18\%$) and so there is little evidence for heterogeneity between studies.

Since the outcome is a relative risk, the confidence intervals for the outcome are calculated on a logarithmic (log) scale and are not symmetric about the estimate. (The same applies if the outcome is an odd ratio.) For example, the RR for the Schreiber trial is 1.20 with 95% CI 0.84 to 1.71. It is easier to fit these confidence intervals on the graph if a log scale is used. However, even then there may be small studies, such as Vento, which has wide confidence limits that would not easily fit onto a sensible scale. The ends of these confidence intervals have an arrow to show that the confidence interval extends beyond the graph. The actual numbers are given on the right of the plot.

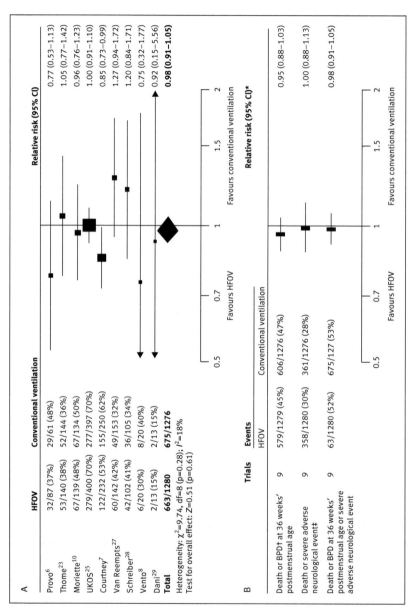

Figure 13.3 Forest plot displaying the results of a meta-analysis of studies with a binary outcome; note that the superscript numbers alongside the author names indicate the original primary papers which are listed in full in Cools et al. 2010

Reprinted from *The Lancet*, 375, 9731, Cools F, Askie L, Offriga M, Asselin JM, Calvert SA, Courtney SE et al., Elective high-frequency oscillatory ventilation versus conventional ventilation in preterm infants: a meta-analysis of individual patient data, pp. 2082–2091. Copyright 2010, with permission from Elsevier

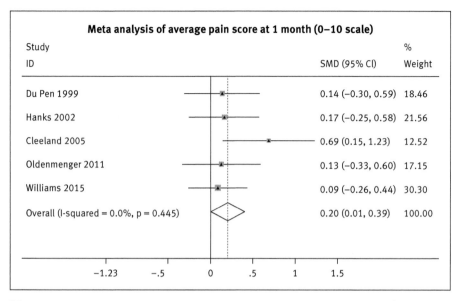

Figure 13.4 Forest plot displaying the results of a meta-analysis of studies with a continuous outcome

In order to help the reader with interpretation of the graph, especially in understanding the direction of the effect, the words 'Favours HFOV' and 'Favours conventional ventilation' have been added to the graph. Figure 13.3B is a plot combining the results of several meta-analyses on different but related outcomes, death, or bpd; death or severe adverse neurological events; and any of these (i.e. repeating meta-analysis A). This format is useful for presenting different outcomes from the same studies when the main interest is in comparing the outcomes. It saves space compared with presenting three different forest plots.

Note the figure taken from the paper has a typo for 'death or bpd or severe neurological events' for the number of events for HFOV. This is reported as '63/1280 (52%)' and should be 663/1280 (52%) as in A. Typos are occasionally found in publications—here, it is not really ambiguous but it might be in other situations.

Figure 13.4 gives a forest plot for a different and unpublished meta-analysis of five trials investigating different complex interventions for undiagnosed pain in cancer patients. This meta-analysis used published study-level outcomes, i.e. aggregated data. The outcome was a patient-reported pain score which was measured on different scales in different studies so the standardized means score (SMD) was calculated for each study and these used in the analysis. The SMD is the difference between the intervention and control groups divided by the standard deviation of the score. Since the outcome is a mean, the confidence intervals are symmetric.

Sometimes studies in a forest plot are ordered by size of effect and sometimes by date, as in figure 13.4. Where several outcomes are presented on different forest plots in the same review, putting the studies in the same order makes it much easier to compare across outcomes and to identify those studies which are present in one analysis but not in another.

Note this forest plot has been calculated in a different statistical package to the one reported in figure 13.3 and so looks slightly different, but the individual study

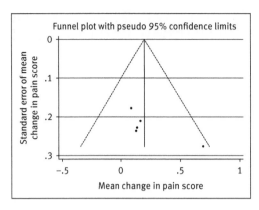

Figure 13.5 Funnel plot to explore publication bias

estimates and 95% CIs are still represented by a solid square and horizontal line, and the overall pooled mean by a diamond—here, open, not solid, but its width still depicts the 95% CI. The plot includes the '% weight' which is used in the calculation of the overall pooled average. The overall average is statistically significant, as shown by the lower limit of the 95% CI that is just above the null value, zero (0.01, 0.39). This shows that, overall, the intervention has a significantly beneficial effect on average pain at one month, although it appears that Cleeland's study has a larger effect than the other four trials.

13.3.11 Risk of bias across studies (checklist items 15, 22)

Statistical methods to test for publication bias are carried out at the outcome level and include bias due to studies remaining unpublished and those that do not report a certain outcome (outcome-reporting bias). Figure 13.5 shows a funnel plot for the data displayed in figure 13.4. If there is no publication bias then the plot should be symmetrical about the vertical line, and no studies should be outside the 'pseudo 95% confidence intervals'. As there are only five studies, it is difficult to draw firm conclusions, and all study estimates are within the 95% confidence limits. The study on the far right is Cleeland's, the one with the largest effect size in figure 13.4. It is possible that this might be an outlier, not necessarily because of publication bias, but perhaps because the intervention, which was a complex one, was not the same in all trials.

13.3.12 Additional analyses (subgroups) (checklist item 23)

Subgroup analyses are analyses conducted on part of the dataset only. They are often conducted because it is hypothesized that an intervention might work better in some subgroups than in others. In the PreVILIG meta-analysis, there was no overall difference in a range of outcomes across the whole dataset and so the collaborative groups specifically sought to determine whether there were any easily defined patient groups in whom one form of ventilation was better. If such a group existed then this would be important for clinical practice. The subgroups chosen were ones where there was a prior reason for believing that a difference might exist—for example, it is known that many outcomes are worse in very preterm baby boys than baby girls born at the same gestational age and

Table 13.3 Examples for PRISMA checklist items relating to subgroup results		EXAMPLE

PreVILIG Study

Item 23

Subgroup analyses of patient characteristics for death or bronchopulmonary dysplasia at 36 weeks postmenstrual age (primary outcome)

	Relative risk (95% CI) (HFOV/CV)	Interaction *P* value
Sex		0.15
Boys (n=1251)	0.89 (0.80 to 0.98)	
Girls (n=1005)	1.00 (0.87 to 1.14)	
Gestational age		0.75
<26 weeks (n=694)	0.96 (0.87 to 1.05)	
26–28 weeks (n=1373)	0.94 (0.84 to 1.05)	
29–31 weeks (n=407)	0.89 (0.60 to 1.30)	
≥32 weeks (n=76)	0.72 (0.32 to 1.64)	
Small-for-gestational-age		>0.99
No (n=1969)	0.93 (0.85 to 1.02)	
Yes (n=286)	0.91 (0.77 to 1.06)	

HFOV: high-frequency oscillatory ventilation; small-for-gestational-age: birthweight below the 10th percentile for gestational age. Fixed effects models are reported.
For further information see Cools F, Askie L, Offriga M, Asselin JM, Calvert SA, Courtney SE et al. Elective high-frequency oscillatory ventilation versus conventional ventilation in preterm infants: a meta-analysis of individual patient data. *Lancet* 2010; 375:2082–2091.

so it would seem sensible to examine the effect of HFOV vs CV by sex since the more vulnerable baby boys might just respond better to HFOV than girls.

To conduct analyses in subgroups, it is necessary to use the whole dataset and fit an interaction term in the model. In the boys versus girls example described in the previous paragraph with HFOV vs CV, this tests the hypothesis that the effect of HFOV vs CV is different in boys than in girls. The interaction *P* value allows us to assess how much evidence there is that the effects truly differ by sex. We can only conclude that the intervention effects differ by sex if the interaction *P* value is statistically significant.

Table 13.3 shows the results of the pre-planned subgroup analyses by sex, gestational age, and small-for-gestation age (a measure of how well-grown the baby is for its gestational age at birth). None of the three subgroups tested were statistically significant (see 'interaction *P* values' in table 13.3). Note that, even though the RR in boys (0.89) is statistically significant, with a 95% CI that is entirely below 1 (0.80, 0.98), and that the RR in girls is not significant (95% CI 0.87, 1.14), this cannot be interpreted as showing that boys and girls respond differently to mode of ventilation. The non-significant interaction test means that the two RRs, 0.89 (boys) and 1.00 (girls), are not significantly different from each other. Box 13.8 gives information about subgroup analyses and notes that these points apply to all subgroup analyses and not just meta-analyses.

Box 13.8 Subgroup analyses   *INFORMATION*

What are subgroup analyses?

♦ These are when separate analyses are done in a part of the whole dataset

♦ They can be **pre-planned** (or 'a priori'), meaning that the researchers documented that these would be conducted before any other analyses are done. Typically, subgroup analyses are documented in a protocol or statistical analysis plan.

♦ They can be **unplanned** (or 'post-hoc'), meaning that a decision was taken to do an analysis in a particular subgroup after the planned main analyses were conducted and seen.Unplanned subgroup analyses may be done to explore the main results in more depth, in which case this should be clearly stated and should be interpreted with care. In other situations, researchers may conduct many unplanned subgroup analyses, perhaps searching for a subgroup where the intervention works. This approach is problematic since the chance of obtaining a spuriously significant finding increases with the number of analyses conducted. If you look for long enough for a significant result, in the end you will find one!

Statistical approaches to subgroup analyses

♦ Suppose we were interested in whether the infants' response to the type of ventilation was different in boys and girls. In other words, is there a difference between the sexes?

♦ This question should be answered using an **interaction test** which tells us whether the effect of the type of ventilation on the main outcome is different in boys and girls. This is the analysis that has been used in table 13.3 and it shows that the interaction test for sex is not significant ($P = 0.15$).

♦ *Note 1*: The RR for males is statistically significant on its own, as shown by the 95% CI that does not cross 1, whereas the RR for females is not. However, the non-significant interaction test shows us that **the difference between these two RRs is not significant** and so it's not correct to conclude that the effects of ventilation differ between boys and girls.

♦ *Note 2*: It is not good statistical practice to do separate analyses in boys and girls even if the subgroup analysis is pre-planned.

♦ *Note 3*: The need to use an interaction test to analyse subgroups applies to other study types and not just for meta-analyses as shown here. For example, in a randomized controlled trial, if we wanted to know if the intervention worked in a particular subgroup but not in others, an interaction test is used to test this hypothesis, as in figure 12.3.

13.4 **Reviewing meta-analyses**

This chapter has focussed on how to report a meta-analysis, as presentation is the main purpose of this book. However, the issues raised are useful to bear in mind when reviewing evidence from a meta-analysis reported by another researcher. Box 13.9 gives helpful tips for reviewing meta-analyses.

Box 13.9 Helpful tips when reviewing meta-analyses *HELPFUL TIPS*

* Is the meta-analysis research question clear?
* Have all relevant studies been identified, including those not published in English?
* Are the study populations and interventions (if trials) or exposures (cohort or case/control studies) clearly defined and uniform?
* Is there any evidence of problems due to publication bias and/or outcome-reporting bias?
* Have the authors considered and if necessary accounted for study quality?
* Has any heterogeneity been discussed and if necessary accounted for using subgroup analyses?
* Is the reporting of results clear and appropriate for the data?

Box 13.10 Further reading *INFORMATION*

Chapters on meta-analysis—give a good overview

* Bland 2015 (chapter 17)
* Peacock and Peacock 2011 (chapter 13)

Books on meta-analyses—provide a detailed description

* Borenstein et al. 2009 (textbook)
* Sutton et al. 2000 (textbook)
* Egger et al. 2001 (textbook)
* Sterne 2009 (Stata guide)

Cochrane website—provides a vast amount of information (http://www.cochrane.org)

* Includes a comprehensive 'Reviewers' handbook'
* Open access to all Cochrane reviews
* Links to all Cochrane groups

13.5 Further reading

This chapter has provided a guide to the presentation of the results of meta-analyses in reports and papers. We also include key points about meta-analyses in general to set the scene but a detailed description of the subject is not possible here. The references in box 13.10 help plug the gap and provide additional reading for readers who may want to see more.

Box 13.11 Presenting a meta-analysis or systematic review   *CHAPTER SUMMARY*

Prepare a detailed protocol before starting and follow the PRISMA guidelines for reporting a meta-analysis. In particular:

- Ensure the study is clearly reported as a meta-analysis so that it is indexed as a meta-analysis
- Describe the eligibility criteria, search strategy, and sources of information. Include a flow diagram.
- Describe the methods to assess the risk of bias including study quality, publication bias, and selection bias
- Describe the data extracted and the methods used to calculate the pooled estimates
- Present the final results as a forest plot including as assessment of heterogeneity
- Present the pre-planned subgroup analyses and include statistical tests for subgroup effects
- Present any post-hoc subgroup analyses openly and interpret findings with caution

REFERENCES

Allison PD. Survival analysis using SAS: a practical guide. 2nd ed. Cary, North Carolina: SAS Institute Inc.; 2010.

Altman DG. Practical statistics for medical research. 1st ed. London: Chapman and Hall; 1991.

Altman DG, Bland JM. Diagnostic tests 3: receiver operating characteristic plots. BMJ 1994; 309:188.

Altman DG, Machin D, Bryant TN, Gardner MJ (eds). Statistics with confidence. 2nd ed. London: BMJ Books; 2000.

Altman DG, Simera I, Hoey J, Moher D, Schulz K. EQUATOR: reporting guidelines for health research. Lancet 2008 371:1149–1150.

Anderson HR, Ayres JG, Sturdy PM, Bland JM, Butland BK, Peckitt C et al. Bronchodilator treatment and deaths from asthma: case-control study. BMJ 2005; 330:117–123.

Armitage P, Berry G, Matthews JNS. Statistical methods in medical research. 4th ed. Oxford: Blackwell Science; 2002.

Barber J, Thompson S. Multiple regression of cost data: use of generalized linear models. J Health Serv Res Policy 2004; 9:197–204.

Barnes PM, Price L, Maddocks A, Lyons RA, Nash P, McCabe M. Unnecessary school absence after minor injury: case-control study. BMJ 2001; 323:1034–1035.

Begg C, Cho M, Eastwood S, Horton R, Moher D, Olkin I et al. Improving the quality of reporting of randomized controlled trials. The CONSORT statement. JAMA 1996; 276:637–639.

Bhat RY, Hannam S, Pressler R, Rafferty GF, Peacock JL, Greenough A. Effect of prone and supine position on sleep, apneas, and arousal in perterm infants. Pediatrics 2006; 118:101–107.

Bland JM, Altman DG. Multiple significance tests: the Bonferroni method. BMJ 1995; 310:170.

Bland M. An introduction to medical statistics. 4th ed. Oxford: Oxford University Press; 2015.

Bland M, Peacock J. Statistical questions in evidence-based medicine. Oxford: Oxford University Press; 2000.

Bolliger CT, Zellweger JP, Danielsson T, van Biljon, X, Robidou A, Westin A et al. Smoking reduction with oral nicotine inhalers: double blind, randomised clinical trial of efficacy and safety. BMJ 2000; 321:329–333.

Borenstein M, Hedges LV, Higgins JPT, Rothstein HR. Introduction to meta-analysis. Chichester: Wiley; 2009.

Bray EP, Holder R, Mant J, McManus RJ. Does self-monitoring reduce blood pressure? Meta-analysis with meta-regression of randomized controlled trials. Ann Med 2010; 42:371–386.

Brooke OG, Anderson HR, Bland JM, Peacock JL, Stewart CM. Effects on birth weight of smoking, alcohol, caffeine, socioeconomic factors, and psychosocial stress. BMJ 1989; 298:795–801.

Bruce M, Peacock JL, Iverson A, Wolfe C. Hepatitis B and HIV antenatal screening 2: user survey. Br J Midwifery 2001; 9:640–645.

Campbell MJ. Statistics at square two: understanding modern statistical applications in medicine. 2nd ed. London: BMJ Books; 2006.

Campbell MJ, Swinscow TDV. Statistics at square one. 11th ed. London: BMJ Books; 2009.

Campbell MK, Piaggio G, Elbourne DR, Altman DG. CONSORT 2010 statement: extension to cluster randomised trials. BMJ 2012; 345:e5661

Cappuccio FP, Cook DG, Atkinson RW, Strazzullo P. Prevalence, detection, and management of cardiovascular risk factors in different ethnic groups in south London. Heart 1997; 78:555–563.

Cleeland CS, Portenoy RK, Rue M, Mendoza TR, Weller E, Payne R et al. Does an oral analgesic protocol improve pain control for patients with cancer? An intergroup study coordinated by the Eastern Cooperative Oncology Group. Ann Oncol 2005; 16:972–980.

Collett D. Modelling survival data in medical research. 2nd ed. London: Chapman and Hall; 2003.

Connor J, Norton R, Ameratunga S, Robinson E, Civil I, Dunn R et al. Driver sleepiness and risk of serious injury to car occupants: population based case control study. BMJ 2002; 324:1125.

Cook DG, Peacock JL, Feyerabend C, Carey IM, Jarvis MJ, Anderson HR et al. Relation of caffeine intake and blood caffeine concentrations during pregnancy to fetal growth: prospective population based study. BMJ 1996; 313:1358–1362.

Cools F, Askie L, Offriga M, Asselin JM, Calvert SA, Courtney SE et al. Elective high-frequency oscillatory ventilation versus conventional ventilation in preterm infants: a meta-analysis of individual patient data. Lancet 2010; 375:2082–2091.

Cools F, Askie LM, Offriga M, and the Prevention of Ventilator Induced Lung Injury collaborative study Group (PreVILIG Collaboration). Study Protocol. Elective high-frequency oscillatory ventilation in preterm infants with respiratory distress syndrome: an individual patient data meta-analysis. BMC Pediatrics 2009; 9:33.

Cornelius VR, Sauzet O, Williams JE, Ayis S, Farquhar-Smith P, Ross JR et al. Adverse event reporting in randomized controlled trials of neuropathic pain: considerations for future practice. Pain 2013; 154:213–220.

Davies HT, Crombie IK, Tavakoli M. When can odds ratios mislead? BMJ 1998; 316:989–991.

Donner A, Klar N. Design and analysis of cluster randomization trials in health research. London: Arnold; 2000.

Du Pen SL, Du Pen AR, Polissar N, Hansberry J, Miller Kraybill B, Stillman M et al. Implementing guidelines for cancer pain management: results of a randomized controlled clinical trial. J Clin Oncol 1999; 17:361–370.

Egger M, Davey Smith G, Altman DG. Systematic reviews in health care. 2nd ed. Chatham: BMJ Books; 2001.

Eldridge S. Pragmatic trials in primary health care: what, when and how? Fam Pract 2010; 27:591–592.

Eldridge S, Kerry S. A practical guide to cluster randomized trials in health services research. Chichester: Wiley; 2012.

Greenough A, Limb E, Marston L, Marlow N, Calvert S, Peacock J. Risk factors for respiratory morbidity in infancy after very premature birth. Arch Dis Child Fetal Neonatal Ed 2005; 90:F320-F323.

Hanks GW, Robbins M, Sharp D, Forbes K, Done K, Peters TJ et al. The imPaCT study: a randomised controlled trial to evaluate a hospital palliative care team. Br J Cancer 2002; 87:733–739.

Harris T, Kerry SM, Victor CR, Ekelund U, Woodcock A, Iliffe S et al. A primary care nurse-delivered walking intervention in older adults: PACE (Pedometer Accelerometer Consultation Evaluation)-Lift Cluster Randomised Controlled Trial. PLOS Med 2015; 12:e1001783.

Hawton K, Simkin S, Deeks JJ, O'Connor S, Keen A, Altman DG, et al. Effects of a drug overdose in a television drama on presentations to hospital for self poisoning: time series and questionnaire study. BMJ 1999; 318:972–977.

Hoek G, Brunekreef B, Kosterink P, Van den BR, Hofschreuder P. Effect of ambient ozone on peak expiratory flow of exercising children in the Netherlands. Arch Environ Health 1993; 48:27–32.

Hollis S, Campbell F. What is meant by intention to treat analysis? Survey of published randomised controlled trials. BMJ 1999; 319:670–674.

Hooper R, Froud R, Bremner SA, Perera R, Eldridge S. Cascade diagrams for depicting complex interventions in randomised trials. BMJ 2013; 347:f6681.

Johnson AH, Peacock JL, Greenough A, Marlow N, Limb ES, Marston L et al. High-frequency oscillatory ventilation for the prevention of chronic lung disease of prematurity. N Engl J Med 2002; 347:633–642.

Johnson S, Marlow N, Wolke D, Davidson L, Marston L, O'Hare A et al. Validation of a parent report measure of cognitive development in very preterm infants. Dev Med Child Neurol 2004; 46:389–397.

Kerry S, Hilton S, Patel S, Dundas D, Rink E, Lord J. Routine referral for X-ray for patients presenting with low back pain: is the outcome for patients influenced by GP's referral for plain radiography. Health Technol Assess 2000; 4(20).

Kerry SM, Bland JM. Sample size in cluster randomisation. BMJ 1998(a); 316:549.

Kerry SM, Bland JM. Analysis of a trial randomised in clusters. BMJ 1998(b); 316:54.

Kerry SM, Cappuccio FP, Emmett L, Plange-Rhule J, Eastwood JB. Reducing selection bias in a cluster randomized trial in West African villages. Clin Trials 2005(b); 2:125–129.

Kerry SM, Micah FB, Plange-Rhule J, Eastwood JB, Cappuccio FP. Blood pressure and body mass index in lean rural and semi-urban subjects in West Africa. J Hypertens 2005(a); 23:1645–1651.

Kirkwood BR, Sterne JAC. Essential medical statistics. 2nd ed. Oxford: Blackwell Science; 2003.

Machin D, Campbell MJ, Fayers PM, Pinol A. Sample size tables for clinical studies. 3rd ed. Oxford: Wiley-Blackwell; 2008.

Machin D, Campbell MJ, Walters SJ. Medical statistics: a textbook for the health sciences. 4th ed. Chichester: Wiley; 2007.

Machin D, Cheung YB, Parmar MKB. Survival analysis: a practical approach. 2nd ed. Chichester: Wiley; 2006.

Maindonald J, Braun WJ. Data analysis and graphics using R: an example-based approach. 3rd ed. Cambridge: Cambridge University Press; 2010.

May C, Patel S, Kennedy C, Pollina E, Rafferty GF, Peacock JL, Greenough A. Prediction of bronchopulmonary dysplasia by physiological measurements. Arch Dis Child Fetal Neonatal Ed 2011; 96:F410–416.

Meyer LC, Peacock JL, Bland JM, Anderson HR. Symptoms and health problems in pregnancy: their association with social factors, smoking, alcohol, caffeine and attitude to pregnancy. Paediatr Perinat Epidemiol 1994; 8:145–155.

Miller MA, Kerry SM, Dong Y, Strazzullo P, Cappuccio FP. Association between the Thr715Pro P-selectin gene polymorphism and soluble P-selectin levels in a multiethnic population in South London. Thromb Haemost 2004; 92:1060–1065.

Missouris CG, Kalaitzidis RG, Kerry SM, Cappuccio FP. Predictors of mortality on patients with peripheral vascular disease: a prospective follow-up study. Br J Diabetes Vasc Dis 2004; 4:196–200.

Moher D, Hopewell S, Schulz KF, Montori V, Gøtzsche PC, Devereaux PJ, Elbourne D, Egger M, Altman DG. CONSORT 2010 Explanation and elaboration: updated guidelines for reporting parallel group randomised trials. BMJ 2010; 340:c869.

Moher D, Liberati A, Tetzlaff J, Altman DG, The PRISMA Group. Preferred Reporting Items for Systematic Reviews and Meta-Analyses: The PRISMA statement. BMJ 2009; 339:b2535.

Oakeshott P, Hay P, Hay S, Steinke F, Rink E, Thomas B et al. Detection of Chlamydia trachomatis infection in early pregnancy using self-administered vaginal swabs and first pass urines: a cross-sectional community-based survey. Br J Gen Pract 2002; 52:830–832.

Oakeshott P, Kerry S, Dean S, Cappuccio F. Nurse-led management of hypertension. Br J Gen Pract 2005; 55:53.

Oakeshott P, Kerry S, Hay S, Hay P. Opportunistic screening for chlamydial infection at time of cervical smear testing in general practice: prevalence study. BMJ 1998; 316:351–352.

Oldenmenger WH, Sillevis Smitt PAE, van Montfort CAGM, de Raaf PJ, van der Rijt CCD. A combined pain consultation and pain education program decreases average and current pain and decreases interference in daily life by pain in oncology outpatients: a randomized controlled trial. Pain 2011; 152:2632–2639.

Peacock JL, Bland JM, Anderson HR. Effects on birthweight of alcohol and caffeine consumption in smoking women. J Epidemiol Community Health 1991; 45:159–163.

Peacock JL, Cook DG, Carey IM, Jarvis MJ, Bryant AE, Anderson HR et al. Maternal cotinine level during pregnancy and birthweight for gestational age. Int J Epidemiol 1998; 27:647–656.

Peacock JL, Peacock PJ. The Oxford handbook of medical statistics. Oxford: Oxford University Press; 2011.

Peacock JL, Symonds P, Jackson P, Bremner SA, Scarlett JF, Strachan DP et al. Acute effects of winter air pollution on respiratory function in schoolchildren in southern England. Occup Environ Med 2003; 60:82–89.

Peacock JL, Sauzet O, Ewings SM, Kerry SM. Dichotomizing continuous data while retaining statistical power using a distributional approach. Stat Med 2012; 31:3089–3103.

Peacock PJ, Peacock JL, Victor CR, Chazot C. Changes in the emergency workload of the London Ambulance Service between 1989 and 1999. Emerg Med J 2005; 22:56–59.

Peduzzi P, Concato J, Feinstein AR, Holford TR. Importance of events per independent variable in proportional hazards regression analysis. II. Accuracy and precision of regression estimates. J Clin Epidemiol 1995; 48:1503–1510.

Peduzzi P, Concato J, Kemper E, Holford TR, Feinstein AR. A simulation study of the number of events per variable in logistic regression analysis. J Clin Epidemiol 1996; 49:1373–1379.

Perera R, Henegan C, Yudkin P. Graphical method for depicting randomised trials of complex interventions. BMJ 2007; 334:127–129.

Petrie A, Sabin C. Medical statistics at a glance. 3rd ed. Oxford: Wiley Blackwell; 2009.

Pinto D, Helano B, Rodrigues DS, Papoila AL, Santos I, Caetano PA. An open cluster-randomized, 18-month trial to compare the effectiveness of educational outreach visits with usual guideline dissemination to improve family physician prescribing. Implement Sci 2014; 9:10.

Pocock SJ, Clayton TC, Altman DG. Survival plots of time-to-event outcomes in clinical trials: good practice and pitfalls. Lancet 2002; 359:1686–1689.

Puffer S, Torgerson D, Watson J. Evidence for risk of bias in cluster randomised trials: review of recent trials published in three general medical journals. BMJ 2003; 327:785–789.

Rees JR, Hendricks K, Barry EL, Peacock JL, Mott LA, Sandler RS et al. Vitamin D3 supplementation and upper respiratory tract infections in a randomized, controlled trial. Clin Infect Dis 2013; 57:1384–1392.

Rees JR, Zens MS, Celaya M, Riddle B, Karagas MR, Peacock JL. Survival after squamous cell and basal cell carcinoma of the skin: a retrospective cohort analysis. Int J Cancer. 2015; 137:878–884.

Sauzet O, Peacock JL. Estimating dichotomized outcomes in two groups with unequal variances: a distributional approach. Stat Med 2014; 33:4547–4559.

Schrader H, Stovner LJ, Helde G, Sand T, Bovim G. Prophylactic treatment of migraine with angiotensin converting enzyme inhibitor (lisinopril): randomised, placebo controlled, crossover study. BMJ 2001; 322:19–22.

Schulz KF, Altman DG, Moher D for the CONSORT Group. CONSORT 2010 Statement: updated guidelines for reporting parallel group randomised trials. BMJ 2010; 8:18.

Spence DP, Hotchkiss J, Williams CS, Davies PD. Tuberculosis and poverty. BMJ 1993; 307:759–761.

Steptoe A, Perkins-Porras L, McKay C, Rink E, Hilton S, Cappuccio FP. Behavioural counselling to increase consumption of fruit and vegetables in low income adults: randomised trial. BMJ 2003; 326:855–860.

Sterne JAC, Newton HJ, Cox NJ. Meta-analysis in Stata. An updated collection from the Stata Journal. College Station, TX: Stata Press; 2009.

Stewart G, Ruggles R, Peacock J. The association of self-reported violence at home and health in primary school pupils in West London. J Public Health 2004; 26:19–23.

Sutton AJ, Abrams KR, Jones DR, Sheldon TA, Song F. Methods for meta-analysis in medical research. Chichester: Wiley; 2000.

Thangaratinam S, Rogozińska E, Jolly K, Glinkowski S, Roseboom T, Tomlinson JW et al. Effects of interventions in pregnancy on maternal weight and obstetric outcomes: meta-analysis of randomised evidence. BMJ 2012; 344:e2088.

Thomas MR, Rafferty GF, Limb ES, Peacock JL, Calvert SA, Marlow N et al. Pulmonary function at follow-up of very preterm infants from the United Kingdom oscillation study. Am J Respir Crit Care Med 2004; 169:868–872.

Thompson SG, Barber JA. How should cost data in pragmatic randomised trials be analysed? BMJ 2000; 320:1197–1200.

UK BEAM Trial Team. United Kingdom back pain exercise and manipulation (UK BEAM) randomised trial: effectiveness of physical treatments for back pain in primary care. BMJ 2004; 329:1377–1384.

Walker G, Shostak J. Common statistical methods for clinical research with SAS examples. 3rd edition. Cary, North Carolina: SAS Institute Inc.; 2010.

Williams JE, Peacock JL, Gubbay AN, Kuo PY, Ellard R, Gupta R et al. Routine screening for pain combined with a pain treatment protocol in head and neck cancer: a randomised controlled trial. Br J Anaesth 2015; 115:621–628.

Yu CK, Papageorghiou AT, Boli A, Cacho AM, Nicolaides KH. Screening for pre-eclampsia and fetal growth restriction in twin pregnancies at 23 weeks of gestation by transvaginal uterine artery Doppler. Ultrasound Obstet Gynecol 2002; 20:535–540.

Zivanovic S, Peacock JL, Alcazar-Paris M, Lo J, Lunt A, Marlow N, et al. Late outcomes of a randomized neonatal trial of high frequency oscillation . N Engl J Med 2014; 370:1121–1130.

INDEX

Note: Tables, figures and boxes are indicated by an italic *t*, *f*, and *b* following the page number.

abstract 39–40
  checklist 46*b*
  for conference 46
  CONSORT checklist 174
  journal article, example 41*b*
  structure, example 40*b*
actuarial analysis (life table
    method) 161, 163*b*
adverse events, CONSORT
    checklist 188
aggregate data meta-
    analyses 196–8, 199*b*
  PRISMA statement 202
  data collection 208–9
  summary measures 210
allocation concealment 182
analysis of covariance 134
analysis of variance
  or multiple regression, choice
    between 145–9
  one-way *see* one-way analysis
    of variance
  presenting 59
  two-way 134
analysis plan *see* statistical
    analysis plans
angular transformation 60
ANOVA *see* analysis of variance
approval for research 34–7
  delays/failure in
    obtaining 37*b*, 38
arithmetic mean 80*b*
audit trails 11, 16
  CONSORT checklist 183
  recruitment process,
    describing 51

back-transformation
  Cox regression with one
    predictor variable 169
  geometric mean 60*f*
  paired *t* test 99, 103*f*
  presenting 60
  regression coefficients 129*b*
  two-sample *t* test
    (unpaired) 78, 81*f*

bar charts 58
bias
  design 196*b*
  meta-analyses 196*b*, 199–200
    bias across studies 214
    bias in individual
      studies 209, 209*f*
    presenting 201*b*
  outcome reporting 196*b*, 199
  publication 196*b*, 199,
    214*f*, 214
  recruitment 193
  response *see* non-response
  selection 196*b*, 199
biconf 17*b*, 105, 108*b*
binary variables
  presenting for a poster or talk,
    example 55*f*
  tables and graphs 58
blinding, CONSORT
    checklist 182–3
box and whisker plots
  continuous unpaired
    data 73–4, 73*f*
  more than two groups 75

case-control studies 72
  matched *see* matched
    data: case-control data
  odds ratio 89, 91*b*
  unmatched, example
    writing up 41
categorical data 58
  graphs 56*f*, 58, 58*f*
  presenting for a poster or talk,
    example 56*f*
  tables 58
cause-specific mortality 65
censored observations 162*b*
character data *see*
    non-numeric data
chi-squared test, two
    proportions 82–91, 85*b*
  with continuity correction 85
  estimates of effect 86–8, 88*b*
  extensions 91–2

presenting 83–5, 86*b*, 87*f*
  Stata, example 87*f*
CIPROPORTION 17*b*, 65
110
  conditional odds
    ratio 105, 108*b*
clinical protocol 22, 23*b*
Clinical Trials Units 11
Clinstat 17*b*
cluster randomized trials 174,
    191–3, 192*b*
  CONSORT
    statement 192*b*, 193
  recruitment bias 193
  sample size calculation 32–3
Cochrane
    Collaboration 195, 217*b*
coding 7–9, 8*f*, 9*b*
coding schedule *see* data
    dictionaries
comparison studies
  sample size calculations
    27–30, 29–30*b*, 31*f*, 31*b*,
    32*f*, 33*b*
  two groups *see* two groups,
    comparing
  two means 28–30, 31*b*,
    32*f*, 33*b*
  two proportions 28,
    29–30*b*, 31*f*
computer packages *see* software
conditional odds ratio 112*b*
  calculating 108*b*
  matched case-control
    data 105
conferences 40*b*, 46
Confidence Interval
    Analysis 17*b*
confidence intervals (CIs)
  chi-squared test, two
    proportions 83
  CONSORT checklist 186–7
  correlation 116
  geometric mean,
    calculation 60*f*
  information sources 70*b*

confidence intervals (*Cont.*)
  logistic regression
    with categorical predictor
      variables 153
    presenting unadjusted and
      adjusted odds ratios 158
  matched cohort data 110, 111
  meta-analyses
    forest plots 210, 214
    PRISMA
      statement 210–11, 213
    publication bias 214
  number needed to treat 191
  presenting 50*b*, 59
  prevalence studies 65*f*, 65, 66
  regression 131, 132*f*
  relative risk 88
  sensitivity and
    specificity 68, 70
  Stata, example 65*f*
  two-sample *t* test
    (unpaired) 78
  when to present 59*b*
confidentiality
  data entry 10–13, 12*b*
  Health Insurance
    Portability and
    Accountability Act 35
CONSORT
    checklist 174–89, 175–6*t*
  abstract 174
  ancillary analyses 188, 189*f*
  baseline data 184–6, 186*b*
  blinding 182–3
  example 177–8*b*
  interventions 177–9,
    180*b*, 181*b*
  non-significant results 188
  outcome data 186–8, 187*b*
  outcomes 179–80
  participant flow and
    recruitment details 183–
    4, 184*f*, 185*f*
  participants 177
  randomization 182, 182*b*
  recruitment process,
    describing 49
  reporting harms data 188
  sample size 180–2
  statistical methods 183
  title 174
  trial design 176
CONSORT flowchart 184*f*, 185*f*
CONSORT statement 200
  for cluster randomized
    trials 192*b*, 193

for randomized controlled
    trials 173–4, 174*b*
  extensions 177*b*
continuous data
  graphs 61–2
  paired 98–101
  tables 58–9, 60–1
  text 58–9
  transformed 59–60
  unpaired
    graphical
      presentation 72–5
    two-sample *t* test 75–9
continuous outcomes,
    dichotomizing to give
    proportions 92–4,
    93*b*, 95*b*
  Stata, example 94*f*
correlation 114–23
  comment on results 117–19
  information sources 132*b*
  Kendall's *see* Kendall's rank
    correlation
  Pearson's *see* Pearson's
    correlation coefficient
  presenting 116, 117*b*, 118*b*,
    118*f*, 121*b*
  rank *see* rank correlation
  SAS, example 120*f*
  several variables 116–17,
    120*f*, 121*b*
  Spearman's *see* Spearman's
    rank correlation
  with transformed
    data 119–21, 123*b*
  when to use 115*b*
cost data 80*b*
Cox regression 166–71, 168*b*
  comment on the results 170
  one predictor variable
    presenting 169*f*,
    169–70, 169*b*
    SAS, example 169*f*
  several predictor
    variables 170–1
    presenting, example 171*b*
    SAS, example 170*f*

data analysis 25*b*
data checking 14–15
  examples 14*f*, 15*f*
data cleaning 14–15
data collection 6–7
  existing datasets 6, 7*b*
  meta-analyses 208–9
  PRISMA statement 208–9

research protocol 25*b*
scanned forms 13, 13*f*
too much data 7*b*
data dictionaries 10, 20*b*
  example 11*t*
  variable names 13
data-driven analysis 34
data entry 7–14
  coding 7–9, 8*f*, 9*b*
  documentation 10
  layout, example 8*f*
  missing data 9–10
  protecting patients'
    information 10–13, 12*b*
  spreadsheets 8*f*, 12
data processing 25*b*
Data Protection Act (UK) 35
data sharing 35, 37
decimal places 49–50, 50*b*
design bias 196*b*
diagnostic studies 66–8
discussion section 45–6
  checklist 47*b*
  statistical issues 45*b*, 45
dissertations 52
  graphical presentation of
    continuous data 61
distributional approach,
    dichotomizing
    continuous
    outcomes 93*b*
documentation 10
dot plots
  continuous unpaired
    data 74, 75*f*
  more than two groups 75
double entry 14
dual approach, dichotomizing
    continuous
    outcomes 93*b*

Epi-Info 2, 16, 17*b*
  comparing two means,
    sample size
    calculation 28
  comparing two proportions,
    sample size
    calculation 28
  prevalence studies, sample
    size calculations 28*f*
  sample size calculations 27
  unequal size groups, sample
    size calculation 31
EQUATOR 1, 193
  data collection guidelines 6
ethical approval 35, 38

delays, common reasons
    for 37*b*
European Medicines Agency 34
Excel
    CIPROPORTION 65
    data entry 12
    graphs, drawing 56–7
    ODDSRATIOANDRR 88
    REDCap 11
extreme values *see* outliers

failed applications 38
feasibility studies 34
Fisher's exact test 85, 92
    Stata, example 87*f*
fixed effects
        meta-analyses 200, 201*b*
    PRISMA statement 210
Food and Drug Administration
    (FDA) 34
forest plots 201*b*, 210–14,
    212–13*f*
    subgroup analyses 188
funding *see* research funding
funnel plots 201*b*, 214*f*

G*Power 2, 16, 17*b*
    comparing two means, sample
        size calculation 28, 32*f*
    comparing two proportions,
        sample size
        calculation 28
    sample size calculations 27
    subgroup and multifactorial
        analyses, sample size
        calculations 32
    unequal size groups, sample
        size calculation 31
geometric mean
    back-transformed data 60
    confidence intervals 59*b*, 60*f*
    paired *t* test 99, 103*f*
    Stata 60*f*
    two-sample *t* test
        (unpaired) 80*b*
graphs
    binary variables 58
    categorical data 56*f*, 58, 58*f*
    continuous data 61–2
    unpaired 72–5, 73*f*
    distribution with a
        cut-off 61, 62*f*
    drawing 56–7
    guidelines 55, 56*b*
    meta-analyses 201*b*
    for a paper 52

population
    pyramids 61–2, 62*f*
    for a poster or talk 53,
        55–6*f*, 58*f*
    referring to in text 57
    two groups, examples 73–5*f*

harms data, CONSORT
    checklist 188
hazard ratio 167, 168*b*, 169–70
Health Insurance Portability
    and Accountability Act
    (HIPAA, USA) 35
heterogeneity between
    studies 200, 201*b*
histograms 61
    before and after log
        transformation,
        examples 79*f*, 102*f*
    checking for Normality,
        example 77*f*
    distribution with a cut-off 62*f*
    two groups on one
        graph 72, 73*f*

I² 201*b*
    PRISMA statement 211
individual patient data (IPD)
        meta-analyses 196–8, 199*b*
    PRISMA statement 200–2
    data collection 209
    summary measures 210
statistical methods and
    terms 201*b*
Institutional Review Boards
    (IRBs) 34, 35
intention-to-treat
    analysis 189–91
    example 190*b*
interaction test 216*b*
interquartile range (IQR)
    box and whisker plots 73–4
    CONSORT checklist 186
    Mann–Whitney *U* test 80
    non-Normal paired data 103
    presenting 58
    rank correlation 123
intraclass correlation
    coefficient 192*b*
introduction section 40
    checklist 46*b*

journal papers *see* papers

Kaplan–Meier survival
    curves 162–4, 163*b*, 165

Cox regression with several
    predictor variables 171
    information sources 172*b*
    with logrank test 164*f*
    plotted upwards
        example 165*f*
    presenting,
        example 166*b*, 167*f*
    R, example 164*f*
Kendall's rank correlation 114,
    115*b*, 121, 12*b*
    presenting 118*b*, 123, 124*f*
Kruskal–Wallis analysis of
    variance 139–40

letters, research 46
life table method 161, 163*b*
linear regression *see*
    regression: simple linear
log file 20*b*, 20
    Stata, example 15*f*
log Normal distribution 60
log odds ratio 153*b*
log transformations
    correlation 120
    paired *t* test 98–9, 102*f*,
        103*b*, 104*b*
    presenting 59–60
    regression coefficient
        129–30*b*, 130–1
    two-sample *t* test
        (unpaired) 77–8,
        79*f*, 80*b*
logistic regression 134,
    149–58, 152*b*
    with categorical predictor
        variables 152–4, 156*b*,
        157*f*, 158*b*
    information sources 159*b*
    interpretation of
        coefficients 153*b*
    preliminary presentation 135
    presenting 152, 155*b*
    unadjusted and adjusted
        odds ratios 156–8, 159*b*
    SPSS, example 154*f*
    when to use 135*b*
logrank test 165–6, 168*b*
    R, example 164*f*
    Stata, example 167*f*
longitudinal research 10

Mann–Whitney *U*
    test 79–80, 83*b*
    and Kruskal–Wallis analysis
        of variance 139, 140

Mann–Whitney U test (*Cont.*)
  presenting 59, 85*b*
  Stata, example 84*f*
  survival analysis 161
manual of operations *see*
    research protocol
masking, CONSORT
    checklist 182–3
matched data 97
  case-control data 97, 98*b*,
    104–8, 111*b*
    information sources 112*b*
    presentation 105–6, 109*b*
    Stata, example 107*f*
    see also conditional
      odds ratio
  cohort data 108–11, 111*b*
    presenting 111, 111–12*b*
    SAS, example 110*f*
  information sources 112*b*
  types 98*b*
  see also paired data; Wilcoxon
    matched pairs test
McNemar's test 105, 107*b*
  information sources 112*b*
  matched cohort data 109,
    110*f*, 111, 112*b*
  SAS, example 110*f*
  Stata 111
mean
  arithmetic 80*b*
  comparison of two means
    28–30, 31*b*, 32*f*, 33*b*
  geometric *see* geometric mean
  multifactorial analyses 135
  paired t test 98
  presenting 49, 50, 50*b*, 58, 59
  two-sample t test
    (unpaired) 75–6
median
  CONSORT checklist 186
  Kruskal–Wallis analysis of
    variance 140
  Mann–Whitney U test 80
  multifactorial analyses 135
  non-Normal paired
    data 102, 103
  presenting 58, 59
  rank correlation 123
Medicines and Healthcare
    products Regulatory
    Agency (MHRA) 34
meta-analyses 195, 196*b*
  aggregate data versus
    individual patient
    data 196–9

bias 196*b*, 199–200
flow diagram 208*f*
information sources 217*b*
presenting 218*b*
PRISMA statement 200–16
research question 195–6
reviewing 216, 217*b*
statistics 200, 201*b*
methods section 40–3
  checklist 46*b*
  describing statistical
    methods 42–3, 44*b*
  example 42*b*
Microsoft Excel *see* Excel
Microsoft PowerPoint 56
Microsoft Word 56
missing data
  data entry 9–10
  information sources 159*b*
  intention-to-treat
    analysis 190
  multifactorial analyses 135–6
  writing up a research
    study 44
multifactorial analyses 134
  information sources 159*b*
  logistic regression 149–58
  missing data 135–6
  multiple regression 140–9
  one-way analysis of
    variance 136–40
  planning 134
  preliminary
    presentation 134–5
  presenting 160*b*
multiple hypothesis tests 7*b*
multiple regression 101, 134,
    140–9, 141*b*
  or analysis of variance, choice
    between 145–9
  with categorical
    variables 143–5,
    146*f*, 147–8*b*
  coefficients 145*b*
  information sources 159*b*
  presenting 59, 141–3, 144*b*
    unadjusted and adjusted
    estimates 149,
    150*b*, 151*f*
  R, example 142–3*f*
  when to use 135*b*

negative predictive value 70
NHS Digital 37
nomogram 26
non-Normal data 102–3

non-numeric data
  coding 7–8
  Excel 12
non-parametric tests 103
non-response
  assessing 51–2, 52*b*
  describing 51*b*
non-significant results,
    CONSORT
    checklist 188
Normal plots 61
nQuery Advisor 27
number needed to treat
    (NNT) 191*b*, 191
  CONSORT checklist 187
  example 190*b*
numeric data
  coding 7
  presenting 48–9, 50*b*

odds ratio 89–91, 96*b*
  conditional *see* conditional
    odds ratio
  logistic regression 135,
    149–51, 152, 153*b*
    with categorical predictor
    variables 153, 158*b*
  presenting
    unadjusted and adjusted
    odds ratios 156–8,
    158*b*, 159*b*
  matched case-control
    data 106, 108
  matched cohort data 111
  meta-analyses 211
  paired *see* conditional
    odds ratio
  presenting, example 91*b*
  SAS, example 90*f*
  when to use 88*b*
ODDSRATIOANDRR 88
one-way analysis of
    variance 134,
    136–40, 137*b*
  further analyses 139
  information sources 159*b*
  Kruskal–Wallis 139–40
  presenting 137, 140*b*
  reference categories 137
  SAS, example 138–9*f*
  when to use 135*b*
oral presentations *see* talks
outcome reporting
    bias 196*b*, 199
outliers
  box and whisker plots 73–4

data checking and
  cleaning 14
graphs 61
overlapping density plot 72, 73f

P values 49, 50b
paired data 97, 113b
  information sources 112b
  non-Normal 102–3
  see also matched data;
    paired t test
paired odds ratio see conditional
    odds ratio
paired t test 98–101, 99b
  back-transformation 99, 103f
  information sources 112b
  log transformations 98–9,
    102f, 103b, 104b
  presenting 98, 101b
  SAS, example 100f
papers 52
  abstracts 40b, 41b
  graphs 52
  tables 52, 54b
partial correlation
  coefficient 123
PASS 27
Pearson's correlation
  coefficient 114,
    115b, 116
  extending the analysis 123
  presenting 116, 117b
  R, example 116f, 118f
percentages
  categorical data 58
  presenting 50, 50b
perinatal mortality,
  presenting 65
PICOS method 195–6, 197–8b
placebos, CONSORT
  checklist 177
pooled estimates 201b
population pyramids 61–2, 62f
positive predictive value 70
post hoc analyses 34
  CONSORT checklist 188
  meta-analyses 208
  subgroup analyses 216b
posters 53–5
  graphs 53, 55, 55–6b, 58f
  tables 53
PowerPoint 56
pragmatic trials 174
  cluster trials 193
  CONSORT checklist 179
predictor variables

area under the ROC curve 70
in logistic regression
  binary 149, 153b, 156b
  categorical 153b, 152–4,
    156b, 157f, 158b
  continuous 151, 152, 153b
in multiple regression
  binary 143, 145b
  categorical 143–5, 145b,
    146f, 147–8b
  continuous 143, 145b
presenting results 20
prevalence studies 64–6
  presenting 65–6, 66b
  sample size calculations 26
    examples 27b, 28f
  information
    requirements 26b
  Stata, example 65f
PRISMA checklist 203–4t
PRISMA statement 193b,
    200–16, 202b
  additional
    analyses 210, 214–15
  data collection 208–9
  eligibility criteria,
    study selection,
    and information
    sources 208f, 208
  example 205–7b
  protocol and
    registration 202–8
  rationale and objectives 202
  results of individual
    studies 210–14
  risk of bias across studies 214
  risk of bias in individual
    studies 209, 209f
  study
    characteristics 210, 211t
  summary measures 210
  title 202
product-moment correlation
  coefficient see Pearson's
    correlation coefficient
profile of sample see sample
  characteristics
proportions
  chi-squared test 82–98
  comparing two 28, 29–30b,
    31f, 82–95
  dichotomizing continuous
    outcomes to give 92–4,
    93b, 94f, 95b
  odds ratio 89–91
  ordered 91–2

presenting, example 92b
paired
  matched cohort data
    109–10, 110f, 111
  presenting 111b
  risk difference 112b
  see also McNemar's test
presenting 50b, 65, 71b
relative risk 88–9
two unpaired 88b
  see also chi-squared test,
    two proportions
Protected Health
  Information 10, 12b
protocol
  clinical 22, 23b
  research see research protocol
publication bias 196b, 199
  funnel plots 214f

QUORUM statement 200

R 2, 16, 18b
  box and whisker plots 73, 74
  Cox regression with one
    predictor variable 170
  dot plot, example 75f
  graphs, drawing 56
  information sources 19b
  logistic regression with
    categorical predictor
    variables 156b
  multiple
    regression 142–3f, 143
    with categorical
      variables 147b
  Pearson's correlation
    coefficient 116, 116f, 118f
  REDCap 11
  scatterplot for two
    variables 116f
  survival analysis 163b
    Kaplan–Meier survival
      curves 162–3, 164f
  violin plot, example 74f
  Wilcoxon matched pairs
    test 105f
random effects
  meta-analyses 200, 201b
  PRISMA statement 210
randomized controlled trials
  presenting 193, 194b
    cluster randomized
      trials 191–3
    CONSORT
      checklist 173–88

randomized
    controlled trials (*Cont.*)
      intention-to-treat
        analysis 189–91
      see also CONSORT
        checklist
    recruitment process,
      describing 49
    statistical analysis plans 16
    subgroup analyses 216*b*
    survival analysis 162
    unequal size groups 30–1
range
    Kruskal–Wallis analysis of
      variance 140
    multifactorial analyses 135
    non-Normal paired
      data 102, 103
    presenting 58
    survival analysis 162
rank correlation 121, 123*b*
    presenting 123, 124*f*
    SPSS, example 124*f*
rank tests
    multifactorial analyses 135
    presenting 103
    survival analysis 161
rare conditions, screening
    studies for 68–70, 69*b*
receiver operating characteristic
    (ROC) curves 70
    logistic regression 151
reciprocal transformation 60
record keeping 16–20, 20*b*
recruitment bias 193
recruitment process
    describing 49–51, 51*b*, 51*f*
    flowchart, example 51*f*
REDCap 10–11
    data checking 14
reference categories
    categorical variables
      logistic regression 153,
        156*b*, 157*f*, 158*b*
      multiple regression 145*b*,
        145, 146*f*, 147*b*
    one-way analysis of
      variance 137
references 3
regression 114, 124–32
    comment on the results 129
    extending the analysis 132
    information sources 132*b*
    log transformations
      129–30*b*, 130–1

several
    regressions 124–6, 128*b*
    simple linear 114, 126*b*
      prediction 131*b*, 131
      presenting 124, 127*b*, 131*b*
      Stata, example 125*f*
      when to use 115*b*
regression coefficient
    standardized 126–9, 128*b*
    with transformed
      data 129*b*, 130*b*
relative risk (RR) 88–9
    CONSORT checklist 187
    matched case-control
      data 106
    meta-analyses
      forest plots 210
      PRISMA statement 210–11
    presenting 52, 54*b*, 89*b*
    Stata, example 87*f*
    when to use 88*b*
reporting guidelines 193*b*, 193
    see also CONSORT checklist;
      CONSORT statement;
      PRISMA statement
reports 52
    sample characteristics,
      presenting 53*b*
    short 46
research aims 23–4
    primary 24, 24*b*
    redefining, example 23*b*
    secondary 24, 24*b*
Research Ethics Committees
    (RECs) 34
research funding 37*b*
    failure 38
research letters 46
research planning 21*b*
research protocol
    meta-analyses 202–8
    PRISMA statement 202–8
    writing 5
    aims of the study 23–4
    approval process 35–7
    checklist 38*b*
    development cycle 22
    failed applications 38
    reasons for 6*b*
    sample size
      calculations 24–34
    statistical analysis plan 34
    study design 24, 25*b*
    summary 6*b*
    title 22

research question
    defining the 4–5
    examples 5*b*
    meta-analyses 195–6
    PICOS
      method 195–6, 197–8*b*
response bias *see* non-response
results, presenting 20
results section 43–5, 49
    checklist 46*b*
risk difference
    Stata, example 87*f*
    when to use 88*b*
rounding 50*b*

sample characteristics
    describing, examples 42*b*, 43*t*
    presenting, examples 53*b*, 57*b*
sample size
    cluster randomized trials
      32–3, 191–3, 192*b*
    comparing two means 28–30,
      31*b*, 32*f*, 33*b*
    comparing two
      proportions 28,
      29–30*b*, 31*f*
    comparison studies 27–30,
      29–30*b*, 31*f*, 31*b*, 32*f*, 33*b*
    feasibility 34
    multifactorial analyses 32
    presentation 33
    prevalence studies 26,
      26–7*b*, 28*f*
    screening studies
      (sensitivity and
      specificity) 26–7, 29*b*
    software 27
    subgroup analyses 32
    unequal size groups 30–1
    writing up a research
      study 41–2, 42*b*
    CONSORT checklist 180–2
SAS 2, 16, 18*b*
    back-transformation of *t* test
      data 81*f*
    box and whisker plots 73,
      74*f*, 74
    correlations between several
      variables 120*f*
    dichotomizing continuous
      outcomes to give
      proportions 95*b*
    graphs, drawing 56
    information sources 19*b*
    logistic regression 151

with categorical
    variables 156*b*
McNemar's test 110*f*
multiple regression 143
    with categorical
        variables 147*b*
odds ratio 89, 90*f*
one-way analysis of
    variance 138–9*f*
paired *t* test 100*f*
REDCap 11
scatterplots
    several variables 119*f*
    two variables with linear
        regression line 132*f*
survival analysis 163*b*
    Cox regression with
        one predictor
        variable 169*f*, 170
    Cox regression with several
        predictor variables 170*f*
University Edition 2, 18*b*
scatterplots
    correlation 116, 116*f*,
        117, 118*b*
    regression 124, 125*f*
    several variables,
        example 119*f*
    with skewed and transformed
        data 119–20, 122*f*
    two variables with linear
        regression line 132*f*
Scheffé's test 137
scientific report *see* writing up a
    research study
Scientific Review Committees
    (SRCs) 35
screening studies 66–70
    for rare
        conditions 68–70, 69*b*
    sample size calculations 26–7
secondary analysis 7*b*
    see also statistical analysis
selection bias 196*b*, 199
selection of subjects 25*b*
sensitivity analyses
    meta-analyses 210
    sample size
        calculations 26–7, 29*b*
    unequal size groups, sample
        size calculations 31
sensitivity and specificity
    calculating, in Stata 68*f*
    extensions 70
    information sources 70*b*
    presenting 67, 67*b*, 71*b*

rare conditions 68–70, 69*b*
single group studies 66–70
short reports 46
sign test 112*b*
    see also Wilcoxon matched
        pairs test
significant figures 50*b*
simple linear regression *see*
    regression: simple linear
single group studies 64–70
    prevalence 64–6
    sensitivity and
        specificity 66–70
skewed data
    correlation 120
    logarithmic
        transformation 77–8,
        79*f*, 80*b*
software 2, 17–19*b*
    graphs, drawing 56–7
    information sources 16, 19*b*
    sample size
        calculations 26, 27
    using 16
Spearman's rank
    correlation 114, 115*b*,
        121, 123*b*
    presenting 118*b*
specificity *see* sensitivity and
    specificity
SPIRIT 193*b*
spreadsheets
    data entry 12, 13
    example 8*f*
    limitations 16
    see also Excel
SPSS 2, 16, 19*b*
    back-transformation 60, 103*f*
    box and whisker plots 73, 74
    conditional odds
        ratio 105, 108*b*
    confidence intervals 16
    graphs, drawing 56
    histogram before and
        after log
        transformation 102*f*
    information sources 19*b*
    logistic regression 154*f*
        with categorical
            variables 152, 156*b*, 157*f*
    multiple regression 143
        with categorical
            variables 144, 147*b*
    odds ratio 89
    paired *t* test with back-
        transformation 103*f*

prevalence and confidence
    interval calculation 65
rank correlation,
    presenting 123, 124*f*
REDCap 11
relative risk 89
scatterplots
    skewed and transformed
        data 122*f*
    two variables with linear
        regression line 125*f*
    standardized regression
        coefficient 129
survival analysis 163*b*
    Cox regression with one
        predictor variable 170
    life table method 163*b*
two-sample *t* test
    (unpaired) 76, 77*f*
square root transformation 60
standard deviation (SD)
    paired *t* test 98, 99
    presenting 50*b*, 58, 59
    standardized regression
        coefficient 129
    two-sample *t* test
        (unpaired) 75
    when to present 59*b*
standard error (SE)
    paired *t* test 99
    presenting 50*b*, 59
    when to present 59*b*
Standard Operating Procedures
    (SOPs) 23*b*
standardized means score
    (SMD) 213
STARD 193*b*
Stata 2, 16, 18*b*
    analysis of variance 145
    back-transformation 60, 60*f*
    box and whisker plots 73, 74
    chi-squared test, two
        proportions 87*f*
    comparing two means, sample
        size calculation 28
    comparing two proportions,
        sample size
        calculation 31*f*
    data checking 15*f*
    dichotomizing continuous
        outcomes to give
        proportions 94*f*, 95*b*
    graphs, drawing 56
    information sources 19*b*
    log file 15*f*
    log-transformed data 79*f*

Stata (*Cont.*)
  logistic regression
      with categorical
          variables 156*b*
  Mann–Whitney *U* test 84*f*
  matched case-control
      data 104, 105, 107*f*
  matched cohort data 111
  McNemar's test 111
  multiple regression 143, 145
      with categorical
          variables 144, 146*f*, 147*b*
      with unadjusted
          and adjusted
          estimates 149, 151*f*
  odds ratio 89
  prevalence and confidence
      interval calculation 65*f*
  REDCap 11
  regression, simple linear 125*f*
  relative risk 89
  sample size calculations 27
  sensitivity and specificity,
      calculating 68*f*
  subgroup and multifactorial
      analyses, sample size
      calculations 32
  survival analysis 163*b*
      Cox regression with one
          predictor variable 169
      Kaplan–Meier survival
          curves 165*f*, 167*f*, 171
      life table method 163*b*
      logrank test 167*f*
      two-sample *t* test
          (unpaired) 76
  unequal size groups, sample
      size calculation 30–1
statistical analysis
  presenting 63*b*
  primary analysis 36*b*
  secondary analysis 7*b*, 36*b*
statistical analysis plans
      (SAPs) 16, 34, 35*b*
  example 36*b*
  multifactorial analyses 134
statistical methods,
      describing 42–3, 44*b*
statistical significance,
      CONSORT
      checklist 186, 187–8
statistical software *see* software
statisticians 20–1
statistics, use in research 1

Stats Direct 17*b*
STROBE 193*b*
subgroup analyses 216*b*
  CONSORT
      checklist 188, 189*f*
  meta-analyses, PRISMA
      statement 210,
      214–15, 215*t*
survival analysis 161, 162*b*
  Cox regression 166–71
  information sources 172*b*
  Kaplan–Meier survival
      curves 162–4, 165
  logrank test 165–6
  low event rates 164–5
  presenting 172*b*
  study sample
      description 161–2
  see also Cox regression;
      Kaplan–Meier survival
      curves, logrank test
systematic reviews 195
  PICOS method 198*b*
  presenting 218*b*
  PRISMA statement 200–16
  research question 195, 198*b*

t test
  paired *see* paired *t* test
  presenting 59
  survival analysis 161
  two-sample *see* two-sample *t*
      test (unpaired)
tables
  binary variables 58
  categorical data 58
  continuous data 58–9, 60–1
  different data types
      presented in one
      table 60–1, 61*t*
  guidelines 57*b*
  meta-analyses 201*b*
  for a paper 52, 54*b*
  for a poster or talk 53, 55*b*
  referring to in text 57
talks 53–5
  graphs 53, 55, 55–6*b*, 58*f*
  tables 53, 55*b*
TeleForm 13
text
  continuous variables 58–9
  referring to tables and
      graphs 57
theses 52

graphical presentation of
      continuous data 61
time to event data 161, 162*b*
title
  CONSORT checklist 174
  PRISMA statement 202
  of research protocol 22
transformed data
  confidence intervals 59*b*
  correlation 119–21
  information sources 112*b*
  presenting 59–60
  survival analysis 161
  see also correlation;
      regression; *t* test
two groups, comparing 72, 96*b*
  graphical presentation of
      continuous unpaired
      data 72–5
  information sources 96*b*, 96
  Mann–Whitney *U* test 79–80
  proportions 82–95
  two-sample *t* test 75–9
two-sample *t* test
      (unpaired) 75–9, 76*b*
  data analysis 79
  logarithmic
      transformations 77–8,
      79*f*, 80*b*
  presenting 75–7, 77*f*, 78*b*
  SPSS, example 77*f*
  with transformed data 82*b*
two-way analysis of
      variance 134
type 1 errors 45
type of study 25*b*
typos 213

value labels 15*f*
variable names 12–13
  examples 8*f*, 15*f*
variables, relationships
      between 114
  checklist for presenting 133*b*
  correlation 114–23
  regression 124–32
violin plots 74, 74*f*

Weibull regression 161
Wilcoxon matched pairs test 79,
      102–3, 105*b*
  information sources 112*b*
  presenting 106*b*
  R, example 105*f*

within-individual studies 97
Word 56
writing a research protocol
   see research
    protocol: writing
writing up a research study 39

abstract 39–40
  for conference 46
checklist 46*b*
discussion 45–6
introduction 40
methods 40–3

results 43–5
short reports and research
  letters 46
structure 40*b*

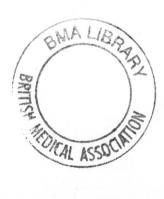